Age Discrimination and the Mandatory Retirement Controversy

Age Discrimination and the Mandatory Retirement Controversy

Martin Lyon Levine

The Johns Hopkins University Press
Baltimore and London

The Johns Hopkins University Press, 701 West 40th Street,
Baltimore, Maryland 21211
The Johns Hopkins Press Ltd., London

The paper used in this publication meets the minimum requirements of American
National Standard for Information Sciences—Permanence of Paper for Printed
Library Materials, ANSI Z39.48-1984.

Library of Congress Cataloging-in-Publication Data

Levine, Martin Lyon, 1939–
    Age discrimination and the mandatory retirement controversy.

    Bibliography: P.
    Includes index.
    1. Aged—Employment. 2. Age discrimination in employment. 3. Retirement,
Mandatory. 4. Gerontology. I. Title.
HD6279.L48   1989   331.3'94   88-9280
ISBN 0-8018-3357-4 (alk. paper)

To Martha, with love

Contents

Foreword

Mandatory retirement is an example of society's use of age as an arbitrary index. Using age in this way may save the time and money needed to make more refined measurements and decisions about individuals, but age-based judgments are often based on outmoded stereotypes that ignore the findings of science or misuse them.

Age is often used as a quick index to the outcomes of aging, by scientists as well as by employers and lawmakers, because it can be useful in grouping information. It is important, however, to distinguish between "age," which is only a chronological marker, and "aging," the underlying, complex set of biological, psychological, and social processes. Not readily to be indexed by age is "competency," the capacity of the individual to meet environmental demands, which is affected by many other factors as well as by aging. It is competency and not chronological age that is of concern to the policymaker.

Research has found wide ranges of individual differences among older adults, though in general they do tend to be slower behaviorally, slower in intellectual performance, less agile, and less physically strong than young adults. Verbal intelligence, on the other hand, remains the same or increases with age.

Four essential facts about aging are apparent in considering the data on age-related competency. First, most of the observed differences may be due to poor health or to disuse rather than to the processes of aging. If we consider a measured behavioral characteristic such as memory or learning, the distribution of these characteristics among active 65-year-olds who are free from diagnosable serious disease is more like the distribution among active, healthy 25-year-olds than it is like the distribution among 65-year-olds who are inactive or have disease.

Second, policymaking must take into account the great diversity and individuality of aging patterns. Some behaviors may improve with age and the individual may become more competent, even though other competences may decrease and the individual may be more vulnerable to dying. Moreover, the differences among individuals will be larger for older persons than for the middle-aged. Chronological age, though it is a better predictor than many other indices of a number of biological processes, is not a good predictor of the competence of the older adult.

Third, while certain competencies of older adults may be limited, research and observation suggest that they may utilize appropriate intellectual strategies, work methods, and concentration of attention to compensate for limitations and losses. Work methods and strategies resulting from older persons' experience may so adequately compensate for the limitations in their component abilities that their effectiveness in their customary environment is greater than it was in their earlier years. This is perhaps most clear in the area of intellectual behavior.

Fourth, because of these adaptive strategies and compensatory work methods, the measurement of decreased component capacities in the laboratory may not be congruent with the actual competence exhibited by the older adult in real-life situations. It is possible for behavioral scientists to measure narrow component abilities with a high degree of precision and reliability, but they are as yet unable to measure the ways these abilities combine to create competence or effective problem solving in real-life situations. If one wishes to assess competence, one must observe the behaviors of people in lifelike circumstances in their ecological niches, allowing for the compensatory functions of wisdom, maturity, and strategies that result in higher levels of competence.

These observations must be taken into account in any analysis of whether mandatory retirement is justified or whether it amounts to age discrimination. One of the special values of Martin Levine's book is the sophisticated manner in which he recognizes these important points about gerontological research.

This book is a landmark contribution to the study of policy issues in social gerontology. Gerontological scholars will find it invaluable in providing new perspectives on fundamental questions on aging. Those who teach gerontology in colleges and graduate schools will welcome the book's well-written and stimulating analysis of the interrelationship of scientific data and policy dilemma. Lawyers and lawmakers will be enlightened by it in rethinking national policies in the light of the graying of the population.

Levine uses mandatory retirement as a case study. By analyzing in multidisciplinary perspective this societal concern, he provides a concrete framework for thinking about issues of intergenerational equity, justice to the aging individual, and a wise response to the aging of the population. His work has value, both for America and for other nations, in considering what decisions should be adopted by private employers, unions, legislatures, courts, and others who help shape social policy.

Levine has succeeded admirably in several major tasks, any one of which alone would be a significant contribution. He has identified and classified what before seemed a bewildering variety of theories offered to explain, justify, or attack mandatory retirement. To do so, he has had to explore a wide range of disciplines important to gerontological policy. He has analyzed and criticized the findings and hypotheses developed within these many disciplines that bear upon the problem of mandatory retirement. Future research on mandatory retirement in particular, and on age discrimination in general, will take as a starting point Levine's contribution.

Competing analyses of mandatory retirement involve a number of empirical claims. Levine has marshaled the data from the various disciplines in a way that makes clear the relevance of research to policy issues. He deals ably with work from economics, history, psychology, psychoanalysis, sociology, biology, and law. He finds that many widely accepted accounts are factually questionable.

But he does not stop there. Levine recognizes that empirical data may undercut certain explanations but that they cannot dictate policy decisions that ultimately require value choices.

If age is commonly used in an arbitrary manner in making policy and program decisions, older adults may be discriminated against, and society's growth potential will be limited by not using their capacities. Discrimination on the basis of age limits the opportunities of the individual, barring him or her from full and equal participation in society. And age discrimination can hurt the community as well as the individual. In her book *Children's Rights and the Wheel of Life*, Elise Boulding argues that the rigidities of age sorting are clearly counterproductive. She adds: "As the world moves toward population equilibrium with declining resources, an aging society will need the fuller participation and wisdom of its elders, as well as the awareness, inventiveness, and energy of its young."

As Levine argues, an aging society needs to rethink how its laws and social practices deal with its elders. Mandatory retirement is an area that clearly raises the issue of the interrelationships between what behavioral scientists know about the elderly, and society's policy decisions. Studying mandatory retirement enables one to understand the controversies over age discrimination, but one must explore the subject with a sensitivity both to the scientific research and to legal institutions. Because of his success in analyzying these complex issues of intergenerational justice, Levine's book is to be highly recommended. It is a most welcome contribution to social gerontology.

James E. Birren
Former Dean and Executive Director,
Ethel Percy Andrus Gerontology Center,
University of Southern California

Foreword

The idea of equality under law is a powerful legal invention. The roots of this legalism run deep, at least in the United States, drawing upon old traditions and the American character itself. There was, of course, a certain logic to the introduction of legal remedies for inequality in America: the law had been central to the maintenance of inequality, and thus only law could undo it.

The idea of achieving equality through law has been an infectious notion too bold to contain. It now has been transplanted across national borders. Moreover, the equality concept has drifted beyond the issue of race, to which it was originally anchored, to embrace a variety of groups. The expansion of the equality idea has been driven by invidious treatment, history, and human progress.

Nevertheless, age discrimination, though perhaps the most pervasive form of discrimination, has lagged behind other types of unequal treatment in the public and even the legal imagination. Only in 1986 was age discrimination in employment barred altogether in the United States, with the historic elimination of mandatory retirement. Thus, a generation after the first modern civil rights legislation—the 1964 Civil Rights Act addressing racial discrimination—age discrimination has finally been put on a par with other forms of invidious treatment. Yet, unlike differential treatment based on race or sex, mandatory retirement, which lies at the heart of the age discrimination quandary, remains a highly ambivalent concept. It continues to have both positive and negative connotations, a unique dichotomy that has impeded the understanding of whether mandatory retirement is discrimination at all. Martin Levine's volume is a pathbreaking contribution to our understanding of this difficult subject.

Until recent decades, we have had little incentive to come to terms with aging, much less with age discrimination. Today medical science and practice, increased access to health care, and increasing understanding of nutrition and exercise have made aging pervasively possible in the developed nations. The same advances, along with nonscientific societal changes, have challenged retirement as a consequence of aging. Thus, scientific and social progress has turned a great nineteenth-century reform on its head. A new set of questions must be asked. Should employment policy ignore or incorporate age? Is age a forced fit with discrimination or is age a status that was merely delayed in finding its rightful place in discrimination doctrine?

To help us confront such questions, Martin Levine provides an unusually ambitious study and analysis that is the most comprehensive yet undertaken. Seldom has an essentially legal question—mandatory retirement—had the benefit of such penetrating interdisciplinary treatment. Martin Levine is at home with the social sciences and with social scientific methodology as few lawyers are today. He pries the subject wide open, refusing to leave it until he has revealed its fullness. His sense of the law of the subject is informed by science, gerontology, psychology, economics, labor relations, sociology, history, and culture. He is not afraid to test theory against empirical fact. He submits law to external tests that can help add integrity and rationality to developing legal doctrine.

Nor does Martin Levine limit himself to the territorial boundaries of his subject matter. His questions are fundamental. Thus, in the process of probing the validity of the age discrimination notion, he brings new understanding to the meaning of discrimination itself.

Martin Levine's rigorous, readable study is particularly important and useful today because so few attempts have been made to discover the core content of the discrimination idea and to test its limits. Even statutes that forbid discrimination generally do not define the term. Someone must. There are jurisdictions in the United States where discrimination theory is applied in the same terms to race and age as it is to the right not to wear a helmet while riding a motorcycle. Without a more rigorous examination of the essential features of discrimination, the salient idea of equality under law one day could become diluted to an essentially political concept without legal or intellectual integrity or, worse, could be trivialized. To ward off such an unhappy possibility, we need strong studies with theoretical and empirical content that are at once careful and far-reaching. That is what Martin Levine has given us.

Eleanor Holmes Norton
Former Chair,
U.S. Equal Employment Opportunities
Commission

Acknowledgments

For their insight into social policy issues of aging and their comments on earlier versions of this book, I thank my colleagues on the faculty of the Andrus Gerontology Center at the University of Southern California, especially James Birren and Pauline Robinson. For their ideas on the legal context of aging, I am grateful to the outstanding attorneys of the National Senior Citizens Law Center and to my fellow officers Cy Brickfield, Eli Cohen, Arthur Flemming, and Charles Schottland. My colleagues at the U.S.C. Law Center are always a source of fraternal support, intellectual stimulation, and invaluable critique; for their comments on the topic and the manuscript I thank them, and particularly Joseph Bankman, Scott H. Bice, Richard Craswell, Alan Schwartz, Larry Simon, Christopher D. Stone, and Jeffrey Strnad. I appreciate the forewords contributed by James E. Birren and Eleanor Holmes Norton.

For valuable advice on earlier drafts or portions of it, or for illuminating conversations, I am indebted also to Bernice Neugarten, of Northwestern University; Richard Cohn, of the University of Wisconsin; Mordehai Mironi and Frances Raday, of Hebrew University of Jerusalem; Shimon Bergman and Jack Habib, of the Brookdale Institute of Gerontology, in Israel; Dan Shnit, of Tel Aviv University; Lawrence M. Friedman, of Stanford University; Carole Haber, of the University of North Carolina, Charlotte; H. L. A. Hart, Ronald Dworkin, Joseph Raz, and John Finnis, of the University of Oxford Faculty of Law, and J. A. Muir Grey and Catherine Oppenheimer, of the University of Oxford Medical Faculty; William Graebner, of the State University of New York at Fredonia; Sally Greengross, of Age Concern, England; and Gavin Brousson, of the Alzheimer's Disease Society, London. I express my appreciation of the late Anna Freud, who graciously made time at Hampstead to share her comments on this topic, to the faculty of the Los Angeles Psychoanalytic Society and Institute who taught me a deeper understanding of the mysteries of the human mind, and to my colleagues on the faculty of U.S.C.'s Department of Psychiatry and the Behavioral Sciences.

Helpful assistance while I wrote the several drafts of this work was provided by my faithful and diligent research assistants Sidford Brown and Minturn Wright; the credit they receive in the text and notes is token recognition that they made substantive as well as technical contributions. Eileen Warburton's painstaking research was an invaluable help in preparing the final draft. I thank also Lisa Kloppenberg for her valuable skills as research assistant, and Renata May for her contributions. The librarians of the Asa V. Call Law Library at U.S.C. were, as always, superb in providing research support. The Law Center word-processing staff patiently dealt with the many revisions; I thank Rachael Andrade, Stacie Dimon-Skotarczyk, Shirly Kennedy, Madeline Paige, Esther Robertson, and Barbara Yost.

Earlier versions of portions of this work have been presented elsewhere. For his early encouragement, I thank Eli Cohen, long-time editor of *The Gerontologist,* where "Four Models for Age/Work Policy Research" was published. "Age Discrimination as a Legal Concept for Analyzing Age-Work Issues" appeared in *Work and Retirement: Policy Issues* (1980), edited by Pauline Ragan, who introduced me to gerontology. A related paper, "Law and Aging," was discussed at the U.S.C. Law Faculty Workshop, where Larry Simon gave a detailed commentary. Some of the normative questions were canvased in "Comments on the Constitutional Law of Age Discrimination," included in the Age Discrimination Symposium supported by the U.S. Administration on Aging, published by the *Chicago-Kent Law Review.* At the Eleventh International Conference of Gerontology in Rome, under the auspices of the Centre International de Gérontologie Sociale, I presented "Normative Justification of Special Rights for the Elderly: Age Discrimination in Employment and Mandatory Retirement," subsequently published in *La Plus de vie* (1986) (in English as *More to Life*). A paper "Is 'Age Discrimination' 'Discrimination'?" was presented at an annual meeting in New Orleans of the Association of American Law Schools Section on Aging and Law. Comments on "Equality and the Elderly" are included in *Justice for the Elderly* (1988), edited by Shimon Bergman and me, incorporating presentations at an international workshop in Jerusalem at the Brookdale Institute of Gerontology, sponsored by the Israel Gerontological Society and the International Society of Aging, Law, and Ethics. A chapter "Age Discrimination: The Law and Its Underlying Policy" appears in Helen Dennis's volume *Age Issues in Management* (1987).

Ronald M. Dworkin graciously invited me to explore these issues with him by coteaching a seminar series in the Oxford University Faculty of Law, "Jurisprudential and Ethical Issues of Aging and Dying." Michael Gelder kindly allowed me to try out my thoughts on aging and law through a number of lectures in the Oxford University Department of Psychiatry to psychiatric and psychogeriatric faculty and staff. And I warmly acknowledge the hospitality of the Master and Fellows of University College, Oxford. As a temporary member of Senior Common Room for 1985/86, I had the opportunity to discuss these ideas with the experts in a vast variety of fields who gather there to enjoy the pleasures of intellectual conversation, high table, and good port.

This work could never have been done without the help and support of my colleague and friend Scott H. Bice, Dean of the U.S.C. Law Center. I thank him sincerely for the many ways in which he has encouraged me. He has successfully created an atmosphere at the Law Center that promotes and facilitates scholarly work. And I thank Wendy Harris, Science Editor at the Johns Hopkins University Press, for her enthusiastic support of the project, and Carolyn Moser for her careful eye and sharp pencil.

The U.P.S. Foundation, the charitable arm of the United Parcel Service, has been most generous in supporting my research as part of its broader program of philanthropy on problems important to society.

About intergenerational relationships I have learned most of all from my son Ben, my father Sam, and my late mother Ruth.

Age Discrimination and the Mandatory Retirement Controversy

Introduction

Is "age discrimination" really "discrimination"? This work addresses the issue of age discrimination through a case study, by examining the mandatory retirement system and its causes. The deprivation of the opportunity to work has been the most widespread and severe disadvantage imposed on people because of old age. If anything is to be considered discrimination against the elderly, the prime candidate for such characterization is the system of age-based involuntary retirement and restrictions on hiring and promotion of the elderly, a system that we can call age-work practices. Age-work practices have been strongly condemned as discriminatory in many quarters, but have also been widely approved by others, who believe them to be consistent with the ideal of nondiscrimination, or even required by it.

Deprivations or limitations based on old age are not limited to employment, but are widespread. Throughout history and across cultures, age has had an influence on determining one's status, rights, and duties. Disadvantages coexist alongside advantages for the elderly. In American law today, age is widely used as a basis for allocating public and private resources, for extending or denying public benefits, for imposing or relaxing legal responsibilities, and for distributing and restricting various types of opportunities. Problems of age discrimination have been recognized by Congress in a number of areas beside employment. And outside the law, there are a number of cultural and social patterns that limit or disadvantage the elderly. Research data show, for example, that the elderly are subject to widespread stereotyping and are typically valued less than younger persons.

The four parts of this work state a problem, review two bodies of studies, and draw empirical and normative conclusions. Part 1 sets out the puzzle to be analyzed, beginning with an introduction to the mandatory retirement system and related age-work practices. Voluntary retirement on adequate income is usually a welcome good, and individually determined involuntary retirement is understandable when a worker's productivity fails. The majority of elderly workers are glad to have the opportunity to retire, and seek the protection of adequate pension and social security systems. But most older persons also wish to protect their right to work if they so choose, and three out of five of the workers who are mandatorily retired want to keep working past the usual retirement age. Justification is required for age-work practices that exclude or

1

retire a worker solely on the basis of chronological age, in the absence of or even in contradiction to individual determination of productivity, and where the denial of a job is perceived by the worker as a substantial harm.

The conventional wisdom on mandatory retirement is that it is both economically rational and fair. It is widely believed, for example, that most people suffer natural deterioration at about the usual age of retirement, so that they are no longer productive workers but dead wood. (The U.S. Supreme Court in upholding mandatory retirement referred "to the common sense proposition that aging—almost by definition—wears us all down.") To try to make individualized assessments of older workers is thus largely unnecessary, many assume. In any case, so the argument goes, it would be demeaning to them and uncomfortable to the rest of us. Whether or not they are incompetent it is also said that older workers are too expensive. Some argue that, whatever their competence or cost, in all fairness older workers should be displaced to make room for the young. Many personnel managers assume that mandatory retirement is an essential part of an orderly promotion system. And retiring each person at a given age is sometimes justified as a system for distributing scarce jobs in a fair, even egalitarian way, using a principle each person would accept for allocating work and leisure over the lifetime.

The strategy I use in this book rests on my belief that normative issues can profitably be approached through a study of the factual picture. The propriety of mandatory retirement can thus be explored by checking the empirical bases of the conventional wisdom and by examining what circumstances and ideas caused the wide acceptance of the mandatory retirement system. If we can understand the basis of the system, we can better judge its propriety under the antidiscrimination norm, and thus better understand the proper limits of that norm.

The mandatory retirement system, though it may strike us as traditional, is fairly recent in origin. The system of retiring workers at some fixed age began only a century ago, in the late-nineteenth-century railroad industry. Over the last half century, mandatory retirement became a moderately widespread practice in industry and government, forcing large numbers of able and willing older individuals to retire. The hardships and costs of the system were substantial enough that it is worthwhile exploring its economic and ethical justifications. The system was not imposed on the private sector by law, and it was far from universally adopted. The people it forced from their jobs constituted only a tiny part of the total work force because many employees were not covered by the practice, or retired voluntarily, or ceased work because of ill health. And the mandatory retirement system was not monolithic: the personal meaning of retirement is different for each individual, and varies with income, class, and sex.

The age-work practices that require explanation can be defined through a list of characteristics; any proposed explanation can then be tested against the list. For example, many mandatory retirement systems included a self-imposed prohibition on the firm's retaining an employee past the stated retirement age, even if the individual remained an outstanding worker. And sometimes a firm adopted a mandatory retirement system for the purported reason that individualized determination of productivity is impractical, while similar firms—and usually that firm itself—had successful experience with individualized personnel determination. An explanation of age-work practices should explain such seeming paradoxes along with the nonuse of possible alternatives that seem economically more rational.

A bewildering variety of explanations have been offered. What caused mandatory retirement? As an ordering arrangement, four models (or, rather, sets of models) are proposed here. Each embraces a range of causal theories, and there is overlap among them. The first model involves a simple assumption of economic rationality on the part of individual firms: it encompasses the profit-maximizing employer response to the supposedly diminishing productivity of the older worker, to the higher average wage cost of the older worker, to the assumed value of turnover of older workers, or to the costs of individualized determination of a worker's worth. The second model emphasizes macroeconomic factors, such as competition among age groups for scarce jobs (sometimes manifested in union policies), and the economy's varying tolerance for inefficiencies in selection of workers. Intertemporal choice is the key to the third model: it includes the theory that retirement is accepted along with seniority as part of an age-earnings profile that overall is advantageous to both worker and firm. The fourth model is that of attitudinal causes, including several psychological and cultural processes. They include factual stereotyping and cognitive error, hostile feelings and ageism, unconscious ambivalence toward the elderly and what the elderly represent, or preference of workers and managers for routinized decisions and a nonmonitored atmosphere, avoiding the need for individualized judgments on continued productivity.

Parts 2 and 3 of this book review a large sampling of the relevant available research. Some studies important to this topic are empirical, others theoretical; their disciplines include economics, history, psychology and psychoanalysis, sociology, and biology. Some focus on mandatory retirement and some include also nonhiring of the elderly, while others deal more broadly with retirement, or pensions, or participation of the elderly in the work force. Still others deal with the history of the elderly, or attitudes toward them, or the skills of elderly workers, or the nature of biological aging.

I have tried to make what sense I could of these diverse bodies of relevant scientific literature and to draw from them what is material to the social policy and legal issues. This survey of the research may be helpful to others, quite apart from the conclusions I draw from it. Gerontologists, economists, and other social scientists may not have had occasion to analyze studies outside their own fields. And legal writers, judges, and legislators considering age-work policies—as well as employers—do not seem to have been widely conversant with the relevant data. Law review writers on the topic, for example, too frequently cite other law review writers for what are essentially empirical points. Because a summary and critique of prior research are presented here in some detail, readers are enabled to judge for themselves the strength of the conclusions drawn. I implore experts in the individual research domains for tolerance of my errors in finding, evaluating, and interpreting studies in fields each of which has its own specialists.

Part 2 deals with studies on what caused mandatory retirement, analyzing them in terms of the four types of models set out earlier. In the arrangement I have adopted and in my choice of headings, I have tried to suggest some major themes, but many of the studies suggest several explanations and could be grouped in alternative ways. Some early studies found mandatory retirement to be largely a product of discrimination or irrationality on employers' part. These same studies also found, however, substantively rational reasons older workers might be thought less desirable, because of the assumed degenerative processes of aging or because of the supposed pension costs of an older work force. A group of studies emphasizes the influence of macroeconomic factors on mandatory retirement. They stress the general forces of labor supply and demand—that is, the existence of a labor surplus or the competition of a particular group (like the educated women who were entering the work force). One explanation speaks in terms of society's overall dependency ratio between the employed and those supported. Another concludes that when there are more jobs than workers, rationing rather than market forces govern, and that mandatory retirement is to be understood as a species of job rationing.

In reviewing some of the more recent studies, I consider at some length empirical and theoretical challenges to their conclusions. One well-known modern theory explains mandatory retirement as a product of economically rational behavior by the employer, who is thought to have implicitly adopted an age-earnings profile in which younger workers are underpaid, older ones overpaid, and the very oldest mandatorily retired. Union policy, rather than employer preference, has also been suggested as the prime cause of mandatory retirement practices. Some well-known economists have set out theories of statistical discrimination, arguing that it is sometimes efficient to judge workers by generalizations: using age as a proxy for productivity may be cheaper than making individualized evaluations even if some good workers are lost in the process. Some sociologists and historians who have studied retirement draw a different picture of the causes of the mandatory retirement system. They focus both on macroeconomic trends like industrialization or competitive pressures and on cultural changes in the conception of the social role of the elderly, while differing as to the relative importance of these two kinds of factors. And a survey of personnel managers highlighted the role of mandatory retirement as a backstop for other practices to create vacancies so as to facilitate a system of internal promotions.

Many of the explanations of mandatory retirement involve external empirical assumptions—for example, as to whether older workers really do lose productivity. Part 3 turns to such external assumptions, reviewing studies on aging, older workers, and attitudes toward the elderly. While there is still no scholarly consensus on many important issues, the research findings do question the commonsense assumptions as to the facts. Thus, there is continuing scientific controversy on the nature of aging, but it does seem that the practice of mandatory retirement at 65 lacks a general justification in the supposed natural ravages of the biological aging process.

There have also been a large number of studies on the job performance of older workers and on specific traits of the elderly relevant to their desirability as workers. Drawing generalizations about the findings is difficult, and the studies often manifest methodological problems, but the research reveals the exaggerations and misconceptions in the common belief that most older workers—even healthy ones—suffer a deterioration of skills at 65 that drops them below the minimum standard for employability. Most older workers who want to continue work could be profitably employed. Indeed, many older workers are more productive than many younger ones, and some traits, like verbal intelligence, often continue to improve. Even diminished skills may still be quite good, and other deterioration is easily compensated for (e.g., by using eyeglasses or by allowing self-pacing). By and large, those who are ill know it and want to retire. It also seems likely that determination of which workers should be compulsorily retired could be done efficiently on an individual basis, without the need for an age-based generalization. Most large firms already evaluate their employees individually; in fact, most of the same firms that had age-based mandatory retirement policies had parallel employee evaluation programs independent of retirement decision making. The belief that older workers are generally incompetent is an exaggeration. Some agree with Congressman Pepper, a great champion of the elderly, who explains this exaggeration as a product of an "ageism" similar to racism or sexism. The research conclusion is more limited, though, demonstrating that the elderly are subject to widespread inaccurate stereotypes as to their relative performance—a picture different from those of other isms.

Many large employers think that older workers must be removed to make room for promotion of younger workers. When changes in the law required that mandatory retirement age be postponed five years, however, very few employers reported that the continuation of older workers in employment in fact caused blockages or slowdowns in promotions.

Supplying accurate information about older workers may be enough to change the age-work practices of most employers. Some employers, however, may ignore educational campaigns and resist targeted informal persuasion. Employers who insist on age-work policies even though they are not bona fide occupational qualifications may be suspected of actual prejudice comparable to more familiar types of discrimination.

Part 4 examines how far we have gotten toward a theory of age discrimination. I use the research studies just reviewed to present some of my own analyses, developing in more detail the three types of models of age-work practices that, in differing ways, explain these practices as products of rational, economically efficient behavior. These models use scenarios that emphasize such factors as the shortcomings of older workers, the difficulties and costs of employers' making individualized judgments, the use of retirement to open up promotions, competition from the young, or some implicit wage bargain.

While the evidence is not clearcut, I draw the conclusion that a major part of what caused mandatory retirement were erroneous generalizations and cultural and psychological attitudes. These factors, making up my fourth type of model, are closer to stereotype and bias than they are to economic rationality. The factors include cultural assumptions about justice and fair distribution of resources between generations, and they may also include common forms of irrational thinking. These irrationalities in turn may stem from stereotypes (adverse inaccurate generalizations) based on cognitive error of a sort widespread in intellectual functioning on all topics. Or these limitations may be affect laden and purposive: unconscious hostility and ambivalence of the kind psychoanalysts investigate, relating to thoughts and fears about one's parents or one's own aging and death. And they may also include psychological processes specifically related to the work place, such as a preference for routinized decisions and a nonmonitored atmosphere. Routinized decisions minimize the emotional costs of individualized determinations by doing without particularized, though more accurate, evaluations.

I then consider the normative implication of these conclusions. Description of social practices is not the same as judgment of them: there are limits to the objectivity of research and its interpretation, a further research agenda needs to be carried out, and knowledge does not obviate normative choice. Empirical knowledge is nonetheless a prerequisite to sound evaluation.

Some of the arguments given in support of the mandatory retirement system fall because they do not relate to the practice as it actually exists: for example, whether or not mandatory retirement could be justified if it opened up many jobs for women and minorities, it is not in fact so justified because it does not do so. Mandatory retirement involves less than 1 percent of the work force and so opens up only a small fraction of the total jobs. Nor is forced retirement needed to create vacancies; most older workers retire voluntarily and still do so even though mandatory retirement has been largely outlawed in the United States. Many personnel managers believed that mandatory retirement was useful as a backstop to voluntary retirement, to keep the channels of promotion unclogged. But similar firms that did not use mandatory retirement managed their promotion process without it, and the firms deprived of that practice by recent law have not seen any need to replace it with alternative practices to create more senior vacancies. Other arguments given to support retirement fall because they rest on inaccurate assumptions. For example, aging does not necessarily render most 65-year-olds incompetent for their work, nor is individualized judgment of employees necessarily inefficient.

I conclude from my analysis of the studies that age-work practices largely reflect certain cultural and psychological processes. We must then make an evaluation to see if the practices, thus explained, are normatively satisfying. I must postpone to another work a full exploration of the normative ramification of these conclusions, through a legal and ethical analysis of the claims of the elderly for equality in our society. Only a beginning of that normative analysis can be presented here.

The analysis set out in this work should lead to reevaluations of practices other than mandatory retirement, which is not the only candidate for the label of age discrimination. The ideas of our culture, the patterns of our society, and the formal programs of our government regularly differentiate among individuals by age—sometimes to the benefit of the elderly and sometimes not. The elderly are the subject of widespread factual stereotyping, as well as some prejudice or adverse emotion. Congress has found the elderly to be widely underserved in federal programs, has labeled the wider phenomenon "age discrimination," and has ruled that it is presumptively unlawful.

Once sensitized to the existence of discrimination in age-work practices, we should be on the alert for the possible existence of age discrimination in other areas, where similar causes may function even though evidence is harder to come by. Governmental uses of old age as a criterion outside employment should also be reexamined once we accept the concept of age discrimination. We should reconsider, for example, whether age-based pensions and medical benefits are based on faulty stereotypes of the elderly, or instead are based on valid principles of need, just desert, or intertemporal choice. It is no secret that there is an apparent paradox in rejecting chronological age as a criterion for retirement, but accepting it for benefits.

Similarly, the conclusion that there is discrimination against the elderly suggests we also rethink the propriety of age-based rules for children. Acceptance of the age discrimination concept as a valid extension of the anti-discrimination principle does not mean, however, that age-based practices are never justified, merely that society must reexamine each such familiar practice to decide which have merit and which should be abandoned.

I • The Problem:
Mandatory Retirement as a Case Study of Age Discrimination

In this part, I examine the modern system of age-based retirement and employment practices disadvantaging the elderly, which I name *age-work practices*. Whether these widely accepted practices are economically inefficient or morally unjustified are important policy issues. The related legal and constitutional questions are whether the practices should be prohibited by extending the concept of discrimination to cover a new category of *age discrimination*. Part 1 starts with some examples of apparently unjustified mandatory retirement, and also illustrates claims of ageism outside the realm of employment. The history of mandatory retirement and the related institutions of pensions and social security is then outlined. To suggest the extent of the cost of mandatory retirement, the following sections review data on its contemporary prevalence and its allocation among industries, the personal and social burdens it entails, and some alternative practices that could take its place. In Chapter 3 I specify a list of characteristics of mandatory retirement and non-hiring that any causal explanation should account for. I then construct four types of models to encompass the various theories that attempt to explain the causes of the mandatory retirement system and to justify it. After stating the problem in Part 1, I go on to review the data in Parts 2 and 3 and state my conclusions in Part 4.

1 • Equality and Age-Work Practices

Albert Schweitzer's Chair

The protagonists of some of the major legal cases on mandatory retirement or nonhiring were forced or kept out of jobs by employers using age-based generalizations, even though the individuals themselves were admittedly fit.

One early case concerned an academic chair established by the New York State Legislature, with princely financial support, intended to attract giants in the various scholarly disciplines to New York institutions of higher learning.[1] The chairs in science were named after Albert Einstein, those in the humanities after Albert Schweitzer. Fordham University was designated to have one of these chairs. After a nationwide search for the most qualified moral philosopher, Fordham chose Paul Weiss, who had been Sterling Professor of Philosophy at Yale and later Heffer Professor of Philosophy at Catholic University. The appointment did not go through, however, because the state education department indicated that Professor Weiss was too old; he was approaching 70, and the officials required the appointment of someone under 65.

The philosopher's son, Jonathan Weiss, happened to be an attorney expert in rights of the elderly, and the philosopher brought suit in federal court claiming that these actions constituted discrimination. The court found, nevertheless, that because "advanced age . . . bear[s] some reasonable statistical relationship to diminished capacity," Professor Weiss was "not the victim of an invidious or impermissible discrimination."[2] In other words, it was constitutional to apply to him a presumption that most academics age 70 are unfit, even though he had been found by the university to be the best-qualified available person in the nation. That Weiss was "a metaphysician of reknown" (as the court called him), that many other great figures in philosophy had done outstanding work after age 70, even that Albert Schweitzer himself had done much of his world-famous work after age 70, did not affect the court's reasoning that age limits on philosophers do not amount to discrimination.

Other leading cases have involved more mundane work. Miss Helen Marshall, a senior dietitian for the Southampton and South West Hampshire Health Authority in England, was forced to retire against her wishes when she was 62, for the sole reason that she had passed the "normal retirement age." Wanting to continue work, she fought the case all the way to the European

11

Court of Justice in Luxembourg. In 1986 she won a landmark victory, in which the European Court analyzed her mandatory retirement as sex discrimination, prohibited by European Community law. It did not consider at all whether mandatory retirement is age discrimination, unfair to men as well as women.

Robert Murgia was lieutenant colonel of the Massachusetts state police. He had passed rigorous annual physical examinations, and there was no dispute that his physical and mental health were excellent. Moreover, his work as second-in-command was presumably a desk job. Nevertheless, under state law he was involuntarily retired at age 50, though Massachusetts local police forces and state police in other states apparently had higher age limits. The U.S. Supreme Court in *Massachusetts Board of Retirement v. Murgia* found it constitutionally permissible for the state legislature to apply to Murgia the generalization that men his age were unfit as police officers.[3]

In a subsequent case, *Vance v. Bradley,* Bradley and other Foreign Service officers sued the Secretary of State to challenge the mandatory retirement rule applied to them.[4] These older employees, unlike Murgia, were in a non-uniformed service not involving public safety; the group worked at a variety of desk jobs, and included accountants, attorneys, and embassy staff in London and Paris. The Supreme Court accepted the assumption of Congress that older persons were unfit for such work.

Unlike the European Court in Miss Marshall's case, the American courts did at least consider the theory that mandatory retirement was age discrimination, taking into account the clause of the U.S. Constitution that requires government action to provide equal protection of the laws. But the American courts rejected the constitutionally based age-discrimination claim.

Age-work policies have their major effect, of course, on ordinary workers. For example, a maid who had worked for a dozen years at a large hotel in Phoenix, Arizona, was fired on reaching age 71, even though she had uniformly positive performance ratings up to the time of her firing. She had no pension or other resources and had to fall back on Supplemental Security Income. A school cafeteria worker in South Bend, Indiana, was mandatorily retired at age 70, despite her "immense popularity" with students. She had no other income. There are countless other examples.[5]

The Practices

In the last century, our society has manifested large-scale *age-work effects*— labor policies based on chronological age that disadvantage the elderly. One of these age-work effects has been the mandatory retirement system; others have been hiring bars against the middle-aged and elderly, and differentiation in promotions or other terms and conditions of employment. These policies were not mandated by law, though laws such as Social Security encouraged retirement, and though governments as employers themselves adopted similar age-work policies. There is continuing controversy whether these age-work effects constitute discrimination—that is, whether "discrimination" is an appropriate label to attach to them. And existing alongside such employment practices were others such as union seniority that clearly benefited the elderly.

One becomes an "older worker," according to the pragmatic definition of the International Labor Office, when "simply because of his advancing years, he begins to find difficulty either in doing his work or keeping a job."[6] The employment problems that come with aging are thus of two kinds. An aging employee may have difficulties "doing his work" because he undergoes real changes in capabilities—for example, finding it hard to maintain a rapid work rhythm. But the worker may also have difficulties "keeping a job" because she finds herself forced out of the work market simply on account of age. As the ILO report observed:

> Older men and women capable of useful and productive work, needing to work and ready and anxious to do so, tend to meet with increasing difficulties as they get on in years. . . . They may encounter discrimination on the job. They may lose their jobs altogether. They may find it hard to get any other job or to obtain retraining. They may be faced with rigid hiring limits. They may find that what they have long dreaded is now happening to them and that for all practical purposes they have been tossed on the "human scrap heap" and that no one has much use for them or interest in them.

Of all these age-work practices, mandatory retirement is the most dramatic detriment inflicted on the elderly. It is the focus of this study.

The Legal Puzzle

There are more elderly and a larger proportion of elderly in the population now than ever before in the history of the world, and individuals live longer and have a longer span of healthy, vigorous life than ever before.[7] These unprecedented demographic and health developments require rethinking of traditional customs and concepts that developed in a different reality.[8] Ideas and institutions that developed over millenia to meet human needs may no longer be satisfactory under modern conditions. Among other new issues posed for society and for the law are those concerning age, work, and retirement.

The concept of age discrimination—a "civil rights" approach—has been employed increasingly in recent years to understand these new issues. The concept has been embodied in a series of congressional actions, notably the Age Discrimination in Employment Act and its extensions, which deal with mandatory retirement as well as with such topics as age differentiation in hiring, advertising, and promotion.[9]

The concept is controversial. Discrimination against older workers has been treated somewhat inconsistently by the International Labor Office and other organizations over the last half century.[10] The application of the age-discrimination principle to government programs has been challenged as intellectually incoherent in an influential article by Peter Schuck. Lawrence Friedman's perceptive book finds the rise of legislation on age discrimination in employment to be a surprising major policy shift occuring with relatively little political demand.[11]

Age discrimination as a constitutional concept has been endorsed by a number of law review writers, but the Supreme Court has nevertheless rejected the idea, showing little inclination to analyze age-work issues in terms of age discrimination for constitutional purposes.[12] There is thus still little or no constitutional law of age discrimination. In *Murgia* and *Vance* the Court said that the aged do not have a constitutional right that age-based generalizations be regarded as a "suspect" classification and thus subject to judicial "strict scrutiny." In dramatic contrast to the Supreme Court, Congress, the president, and many of the states have adopted age discrimination as a key concept in dealing with age-work problems.

Whether it is appropriate to apply a legal concept of "age discrimination" to mandatory retirement depends in large part on the causes of the practice. While many people think they have a commonsense explanation for mandatory retirement, based on anecdote and introspection, common sense may be wrong. Mandatory retirement is an economic and historical puzzle: an essential part of the legal analysis is to figure out what the facts are.[13] In developing a law about treatment of the elderly, the starting point should be what we can find out about causes of the treatment of older persons and the actual facts about aging and the elderly,[14] rather than some abstract constitutional formula. Getting a grasp on the real-world problem calling for judgment provides the vital first step in making a normative judgment. It is at least as important as the issues of political theory and constitutional interpretation that delight legal scholars.

The Supreme Court's approach to equal protection issues, as exemplified in the leading age-work case, invokes abstract formula but leaves the way open for renewed attention to real-world facts. The Court's conclusion as to mandatory retirement is: "While the treatment of the aged in this Nation has not been wholly free of discrimination, such persons, unlike, say, those who have been discriminated against on the basis of race or national origin, have not experienced a 'history of purposeful unequal treatment' or been subjected to unique disabilities on the basis of stereotyped characteristics not truly indicative of their abilities."[15]

The employment practices of the private sector are set by management or through collective bargaining, but they are potentially subject to regulation by the legislature on the national or state level. The laws the legislature adopts—including those on public-sector employment practices—are themselves subject to judicial review in the United States to determine if they satisfy the requirements of the U.S. Constitution, including its equal protection clause.

U.S. legislation has endorsed the age-discrimination concept. The original Age Discrimination in Employment Act of 1967 (ADEA) protected workers only up to a cap of age 65. The 1978 ADEA Amendments extended coverage to age 70 in the private sector and to older workers without maximum limit in most government positions.[16] The 1986 ADEA Amendments uncapped the statute's protection in most parts of the private sector.[17] Thus, the current law prohibits the familiar custom of age-based mandatory retirement for most employees of public agencies and large private businesses. Basically, the ADEA prohibits using middle or old age as a personnel criterion, except when age is indeed a "bona fide occupational qualification." In this statute Congress employed an age-discrimination concept, the use of which was justified by some proponents through an explanation of mandatory retirement as a product of intergenerational prejudices. Twenty-four of the fifty states have independently adopted their own bans on age-based mandatory retirement, for public or private sectors or both, and generally without any maximum age limit.[18]

The early Supreme Court cases construing the ADEA seemed unfriendly to its purposes. As one commentator put it:

> Paradoxically, Congress' deliberate movement toward greater protection of the elderly against employment discrimination has met noticeable opposition from segments of the federal judiciary, including the Supreme Court. . . . The conclusion arguably to be derived from the holdings in these [early] cases is that the Court has construed the ADEA and its amendments so narrowly that the broad age discrimination protection Congress intended for the elderly has not been fully realized.[19]

In the landmark equal-protection cases of *Massachusetts Board of Retirement v. Murgia* and *Vance v. Bradley* the Supreme Court rejected the age-discrimination concept in a constitutional context. It sustained as constitutional various mandatory retirement laws for government employees, refusing to extend the antidiscrimination principle to recognize a constitutional concept of age discrimination. The Court did so in part because constitutional equal-protection adjudication has a narrower scope than legislative policy-making. Under the current approach, the Court said: "Equal protection analysis requires strict scrutiny of a legislative classification only when the classification impermissibly interferes with the exercise of a fundamental right or operates to the peculiar disadvantage of a suspect class. Mandatory retirement . . . involves neither situation."[20] But beyond the analytic framework of equal protection doctrine, a central part of the Court's analysis was its apparent explanation of mandatory retirement as an acceptable product of economically rational behavior.[21] In apparent inconsistency, the Court's recent cases interpreting the ADEA appear to adopt the congressional view of mandatory retirement as essentially arbitrary.[22]

In the constitutional cases, the Court's understanding of the institution of mandatory retirement in general was the key to its decision to refuse to scrutinize strictly the particular challenged policies as constitutional violations. A general explanation of mandatory retirement is of special relevance to the key constitutional issue raised by current legal doctrine on the equal protection clause: choosing the so-called level of scrutiny. When deciding a claim under the constitutional guarantee of equal protection of the laws, an American court will first decide which of three tiers of scrutiny to apply. Most laws are judged by an easily met standard of "minimal rationality": they are regarded as presumptively constitutional and will be upheld by the courts as long as the classification employed can somehow be construed as a reasonable means to any legitimate governmental purpose. Only a few legislative classifications (notably those based on race) are instead regarded as "suspect" and accorded judicial "strict scrutiny"; they are presumptively unconstitutional unless they can be shown to be "necessary" to "compelling" or "overriding" social purposes. And a few laws (mostly classifying by sex) are judged under an "intermediate standard." In the cases challenging mandatory retirement, the Supreme Court has thus far ruled that only the lowest (minimal-rationality) level of scrutiny is applicable to age-based laws; almost any law can survive such an undemanding constitutional test. A reexamination of the causes of mandatory retirement is crucial to determining whether these laws should instead be judged by the much harsher standards of strict or intermediate judicial scrutiny under the equal protection clause. The constitutional controversy is thus whether the law should deal with age discrimination as it deals with race and sex discrimination.

If the causes of age-work practices derive from consideration of economic efficiency, they are perhaps more likely to be justifiable: for example, perhaps "rational prejudice"[23] or "statistical discrimination"[24] is not necessarily discrimination in a legal sense. On the other hand, if age-work practices derive from ordinary emotional prejudice (a "taste" for discrimination)[25] they apparently violate society's antidiscrimination norm, unless insulated from it as purely private action. I survey the studies on the causes of age-work practices in Part 2.

A number of writers argue, in effect, that age discrimination in employment is so unlike the race-based or sex-based employment practices we term discrimination that they do not deserve the same label. Thus, Peter Schuck asserts that older workers are unlike true "minority groups" because the elderly are objects of social privileges, not consistently singled out for adverse treatment.[26] A writer in the *Columbia Law Review* argued that "older workers are not subject to the pervasive social stigma and presumption of inferiority historically attached to some groups protected under title VII," which is the general law on employment discrimination based on race, color, religion, sex, and national origin. Therefore, she concludes that older workers "are not in need of the degree of vigilant protection accorded other groups."[27] Similarly, a writer in the *Harvard Law Review* argued that the ADEA is unlike Title VII, because that broader civil rights law—but not the age legislation—serves the comprehensive social function of ameliorating widespread effects of past discrimination and of providing positive role models.[28]

Deciding how the law should deal with mandatory retirement is in turn a testing case for formulating a general legal principle of equality. If we can decide whether age discrimination is a valid analogy to what we normally deem discrimination, we will know better how to deal with claims from others seeking the extension to them of the current legal guarantees of equality.[29] Solving the age-discrimination puzzle would help us approach related issues of discrimination law such as why gender discrimination is given special treatment, and whether similar special treatment should be used to protect other disadvantaged groups.[30]

Some have argued that age discrimination is not really discrimination because it is limited to employment, but it is not in fact so limited. In many cultures age helps determine one's status, rights, and duties.[31] In the United States, age is widely used as a basis for allocating public and private resources, for extending or denying public benefits, for imposing or relaxing legal responsibilities, and for distributing and restricting various types of opportunities.[32] Whether age differentiation is justifiable generally or in specific cases, it is hardly rare for such differentiation to exist and for deprivations or limitations to be based on old age.

There are a number of cultural and social patterns that limit the elderly. The depiction of the elderly in the mass media has been termed ageist, and the scientific data shows that there is widespread stereotyping of the elderly and a relative devaluation of the elderly as compared to younger cohorts.[33] And remembering the famous discriminatory question "Would you want your sister to marry one?" we can recognize that under the cultural expectations and social practices common in our country today, marriage or sexual relations between the elderly and the young are frowned upon.

The concept of age discrimination has been used by Congress in a number of areas beside employment.[34] The existence of such federal statutes shows the opinion of the national legislature that age-based differentiation exists in a wide range of areas and deserves condemnation as unjustified.

Most age-based compulsory retirement rules are presently prohibited by the 1978 and 1986 ADEA Amendments. An explanation of mandatory retirement (say, as a product of discrimination, or of strivings toward efficiency) nevertheless is still important to remaining issues of age-work policy, as governments and firms consider how age-based rules should influence employment practices. Such remaining issues include the following: Should the ADEA be interpreted narrowly, as the Supreme Court initially did, or broadly, as the Court has done in its recent cases? Should the ADEA's remaining exceptions be extended or abolished? Should other countries whose laws reflect a strong antidiscrimination principle, like the United Kingdom, adopt laws against age discrimination in employment? How should Canada apply to employment its new constitutional ban on "age discrimination"? Should the Supreme Court reverse its current attitude (as three Supreme Court justices have hinted)[35] and examine with heightened constitutional scrutiny the few remaining government mandatory retirement rules?[36]

The Conventional Wisdom on Mandatory Retirement

The use of chronological age as a main (or, indeed, as the sole) criterion in personnel decisions, an English scholar has noted, "may seem, in the light of conventional wisdom, wholly reasonable."[37] As put by the columnist William Safire, "Old people get older and usually less productive, and they ought to retire so that business can be better managed and more economically served."[38] The *locus classicus* for that conventional wisdom on older workers is the U.S. Supreme Court. The Court told us in *Murgia* that "physical ability generally declines with age" and that "fitness for uniformed service presumptively has diminished with age."[39] In *Vance* it added that "increasing age brings with it increasing susceptibility to physical difficulties" and mentioned "the common sense proposition that aging—almost by definition—inevitably wears us all down."[40] The Court was informed by various studies and testimony referred to in the record of the cases, but, given that five of its nine members were already over age 70,[41] perhaps the justices were largely influenced by their impressions about themselves, their spouses, their friends, and one another.

The Court in *Vance* seemed convinced of the widespread accuracy of this position, for it uttered its comments about older workers' unsuitability in a case dealing with a variety of desk jobs.[42] Moreover, the case came up to the Supreme Court at a procedural stage where the government must be taken as having admitted as true the affidavits submitted by the plaintiff-workers to demonstrate that most employees in fact continue to be competent.[43] In a later case, *Slate v. Noll,* the Supreme Court went even further: it thought that no written opinion was necessary to extend its position on mandatory retirement to cover all the types of jobs in a state's civil service system.[44]

The sitting Supreme Court justices may think it only "common sense" that we all gradually decline as we grow older. Some scientists, however, think the evidence is more in line with the vision Oliver Wendell Holmes, Sr., expressed in his famous verses on the "one-hoss-shay":

> Have you heard of the wonderful one-hoss-shay
> That was built in such a logical way
> It ran a hundred years to a day
> And then . . .
>
> .   .   .   .
> [I]t went to pieces all at once—
> All at once, and nothing first,
> Just as bubbles do when they burst.[45]

Thus, Fries and Crapo's theory of the "rectangular curve" suggests that, unless there is injury or infection from the outside, human beings may perform close to peak capacity until a last, brief, fatal illness.[46] And James Birren has similarly concluded that "there is the possibility that the psychological norm for the species is one of little change in intellectual function in the years after 65, given good health."[47] These observations concern the human species in general, not any particular group of older workers, but because health-related voluntary retirement is common, the sample of older persons who want to continue working is even healthier than the full population of persons of that age cohort.

The Supreme Court's commonsense proposition can be restated: the process capsulized by the term *aging* is thought to involve changes in older workers at about the typical retirement age so that they commonly fall below the productivity required for continued employment. I call this explanation of mandatory retirement a substantively rational one. Logic seems to require that this proposition include the further steps enunciated by courts interpreting the "bona fide occupational qualification" standard of the Age Discrimination in

Employment Act[48]—either that substantially all older persons fall below that productivity standard or that most do and that individual determination is impractical.[49]

The "commonsense" proposition may be tested against four bodies of research. We would want to know what biological process is referred to by the term *aging*, so that we can tell whether it is true that "almost by definition," it wears us all down. We also need data on the productivity of older workers, and it would also be useful to have studies of the characteristics of older persons relevant to their productivity. (There may be some age, other than the customary 65, when the commonsense generalization about older workers becomes an accurate generalization. Perhaps 75 or 80 is that age and would serve as the dividing line between the "young old" and the "old old.")[50] Finally, we want to know whether or not it is impractical to use individualized determinations of which older persons are, and which are not, sufficiently productive to remain employed. The data on these four topics are explored in Part 3.

2 • Mandatory Retirement and Nonhiring

Retirement as a Historical Institution

Early studies of age-work practices identified such causes as the technological environment and the influence of pensions, group insurance, and workmen's compensation rules. Later studies have highlighted negative stereotypes about older workers as the dominant cause.[1]

The social institution of mandatory retirement at a fixed age may seem to us to be natural and timeless, but it is a phenomenon of the last hundred years, along with the major pension and social security systems. It was not a normal custom in early America. Historically, when workers did retire they did so because of individual circumstances and not because some predetermined age had been reached.[2] The earliest widespread American old-age pension system (overlooked by many scholars) provided pension eligibility outside a retirement system: there were both state and federal pensions for veterans of every American war, notably the pensions for Civil War veterans and their widows won by the Grand Army of the Republic.[3]

In the late nineteenth century, typical work careers were disorderly; even highly skilled workers were forced into temporary jobs in unskilled occupations during the last third of their lives.[4] The idea that workers retire at a fixed age first gained currency in that period. In America, private pensions began in the railroad industry; they were first proposed by the American Express Company in 1875 and first put into effect as a functioning plan by the Baltimore and Ohio Railroad in 1884.[5] A related practice of laying off rather than reassigning slow workers was adopted about 1920, for example, by the Amoskeag Corporation, the world's largest textile manufacturer.[6]

There are also statistical data on prevalence of age-work practices half a century ago, in 1929. As to maximum hiring-age policies, an Equitable Life Assurance survey of 1,600 group-insurance patrons (one-third of whom replied) showed that 60 percent reported no age bars on hiring.[7] In a National Association of Manufacturers survey of "thousands" of its members, 70 percent reported no such hiring limit. "A considerable number of companies reported that they preferred older employees . . . while the investigation disclosed no companies which discharged employees when they reached a given age." Of companies with age limits on hiring, "many" made exceptions for former employees who wished to rejoin them. One-fifth of those with age limits on new hires gave as a reason their wish to maintain plant pension plans and the "special obligation to provide steady employment to those already in their employ for many years."[8] The report does not mention whether pension plans involved mandatory retirement, which might not have been deemed "discharge."

Pensions

Not until the 1940s was there widespread adoption of formal pension plans, and then primarily for executives. Only after World War II did pension coverage gradually spread to ordinary workers, and only then did it become a more important labor-supply trend than reductions in working hours.[9]

Pension systems with a minimum eligibility age were established by firms largely to appease workers and provide some control over them. In addition, older workers were thought to be "used up," and thus firms tended to use the pension eligibility age also as a maximum work age. The pension and mandatory retirement systems were interrelated because the first helped legitimate the second. As unions sought seniority systems, firms had an additional reason to want mandatory retirement: older workers were more expensive, and age-based retirement was a way of limiting the cost of seniority. Furthermore, the impersonal age-based system was simple for large firms to administer. Unions sometimes acquiesced in mandatory retirement as a bargaining trade-off and sometimes sought it as a way of reallocating work: union employees were more than twice as likely to face mandatory retirement as nonunion. Collective bargaining may have contributed to the acceptance of mandatory retirement as part of pension plans. As often as not, bargaining agreements included compulsory retirement provisions. But unionization did not necessarily have a significant effect on the incidence of mandatory retirement.

The general law did not require mandatory retirement, but over time governments, like industry, adopted retirement systems for their own employees.

Social Security

The major Western governments, over the course of half a century, also established national social security provisions. The first national pension system is usually thought to be Bismarck's: Germany adopted its Old Age and Survivors Pension Act in 1889. It initially set the retirement age at 70, far above the average worker's life expectancy, and thus could afford to pay full benefits to the few covered retirees only two years after the system was adopted.

By 1916, the German retirement age was reduced to 65, although life expectancy had increased.[10]

A number of countries introduced national old-age pensions substantially later, in the 1930s and '40s, generally fixing the retirement age at 65. The United States had pensions for civil service employees by 1920 and for railroad workers by 1934. The U.S. national old age system, the Social Security Act, was adopted in 1935, following a decade of political activity by older Americans. The original act passed the House of Representatives with no requirement that old-age-insurance beneficiaries be retired.[11] The *retirement test* was added by the Senate Finance Committee on the rationale that "there is no need for payment of old-age benefits to workers who have reached age 65 but who still continue in regular employment."[12] The act thus encouraged retirement at 65 by providing a pension, by setting a "usual" age, and by applying a retirement test for benefits that was the equivalent of a 50 percent tax rate for continued work between normal retirement age and age 72. With these payments available, many Americans came to view retirement as a reward or benefit.[13]

The literature gives a variety of reasons why the social security and national pension plans were adopted and why specific ages were chosen. Fiscal and political reasons were important for public systems. The initial German age of 70 was so high that total pay-outs would be low, so that the system could afford to start paying benefits to some people quickly. Age 65 enabled more people to qualify for payments, showing the usefulness of pensions in reducing poverty among the elderly. Thus, both ages were chosen in part to increase public support for the systems.[14]

The economic crisis of the Depression evoked a vision of a welfare state.[15] William Graebner speaks of Social Security in the United States as a political response to large-scale unemployment and poverty among the old, as well as a way of rationalizing mandatory retirement and age discrimination in employment.[16] It was a part of a social ideology that justified the federal government's responsibility for managing the economy and providing general social welfare policies.[17] Whatever the original goals of Social Security, as its eligibility and benefits grew, it had major influence in removing workers from the labor force and " 'reducing' unemployment," as Malcolm Morrison puts it.[18]

Additional reasons for the adoption of social security and pension systems include macroeconomic factors and intergroup competition. From the late nineteenth century through the Depression there was a labor surplus, and the retiring of older workers was thought important to open up jobs for young people. Most scholars would agree with Howard, Peavy, and Selden that "it was clear from the beginning that one of . . . [Social Security's] major functions was to encourage older workers to withdraw from the labor force, making more jobs available to younger workers."[19] Intertemporal choice was considered: most people were thought to want more leisure after thirty-five to forty years of work. Supposed substantive rationality was also important. Thus, Tracy says that in fixing the Social Security age at 65, Congress gave consideration to the age at which it was thought that workers tend to lose the ability to keep up with the technological advances of industrial society, are frequently subject to ill health and disability, and are less productive under difficult work conditions.[20] Notwithstanding such beliefs, the large demand for labor during World War II "briefly suspended negative attitudes toward older workers. Thousands were employed with little difficulty, and there were few complaints about performance."[21]

The Contemporary Prevalence of Retirement

Labor-Force Participation

With the increase in life expectancy and healthy lives in our era, there is a large elderly population for the first time in human history.[22] The population age 65 and over is expected to increase from 25 million in 1980 (11% of the population) to 32 million in the year 2000 (13% of the population), using intermediate demographic assumptions.[23] Nevertheless, the normal working life of American men has been shrinking, and the fraction of the male population over 65 who work (the civilian-labor-force participation) has drastically diminished.[24] In 1890 two out of every three older men were in the work force. By 1960 the ratio was one out of three, dropping to one out of five by 1980.[25] The rate dropped nearly twenty points in the two decades after 1957.[26] For men 65–69, fewer than three out of ten remained in the labor force in 1980.[27]

Voluntary individual choices to retire account for much of the trend for older workers to leave the work force early. In one British study, for example, seven out of ten male factory workers in "good" health wanted to retire. Other research suggests that 40 percent of those who are subject to mandatory retirement retire willingly; 20 percent of the cohort reaching usual retirement age have already chosen early retirement.[28]

Workers choose to retire for many individual reasons. Some scholars have speculated that leisure is increasingly a value and the work ethic itself has declined, so that work is now less commonly an end in itself. Other explanations are available.[29] The substantial lowering of the labor-force participation of older workers, along with a trend to early retirement, were supported both by the increasing availability of Social Security and private pension benefits as well as by the influence of mandatory retirement practices.[30] Palmore and associates, in a 1985 book, *Retirement,* found differences by sex, race, and socioeconomic status for causes of retirement.[31] Voluntary retirement was influenced by pension eligibility and provisions, health, family financial obligations, the difficulty of finding satisfactory employment, and the expectation that people retire by the usual age.[32] Most retirement at normal ages, Palmore and his coauthors concluded, is forced or encouraged by mandatory retirement policies and expectations of employers, fellow workers, and family. In contrast, they concluded that most early retirement is neither forced nor expected and is more influenced by perceptions of retirement benefits, health, and work.

Many scholars have emphasized that poor health is an important cause of the decision to retire. In so doing they rely on two bodies of research: surveys of reasons stated by those retiring, and correlation or regression studies showing that poor health is in fact associated with earlier retirement.[33]

The dominant reasons for retirement are usually found to be income-related. Eligibility for retirement on pension adds an opportunity cost to continued work; in the decline of labor-force participation rates among men over 60, the most significant factor is thus the growing financial ability of older men to retire early.[34] Partial explanations of the sharpest drops among males can be explained simply: they occur at ages 62 and 65, the key ages for Social Security benefits, when retirement becomes economically more feasible and the opportunity costs of continuing to work increase.[35] One study calculated that current eligibility for an employer pension lowered the probability of being in the labor force by 9.2 percent in 1973.[36] Gary Fields and Olivia Mitchell, in their 1984 book *Retirement, Pensions, and Social Security,* concluded that economic factors have an important role in the voluntary retirement decision, and that the decision is best understood in an intertemporal (or life-cycle) framework. People consider not only the immediate income and leisure opportunities available if they retire but also take into account the costs and benefits (such as enhanced pension benefits) if they work a few years more. Fields and Mitchell did a statistical calculation using an analysis of variance and concluded that, of the variation in voluntary retirement age that can be explained, economic variables explain about three-quarters and health variables about one-quarter.

The Incidence of Mandatory Retirement

Mandatory retirement practices stand alongside voluntary retirement as a cause of diminished participation by the elderly in the work force. The labor-force participation rate of older men is in large part dependent on the demand for their services (the age-work effect) and not merely the supply (determined by voluntary retirement). Employer exclusion of the elderly from the job market, when not prohibited by government, has accounted for a significant part of the lowered participation rates of the elderly.[37] A landmark 1965 U.S. government report, *The Older American Worker,* documented the fact that in states without protective legislation both applicants for new positions and older workers already on the payroll had been subjected to exclusion from employment opportunity because of widespread mandatory retirement policies and refusal to hire the elderly.[38] Eliminating mandatory retirement was calculated by the Labor Department to have a substantially larger effect on the labor-force participation of older men than removing work disincentives from pensions or cutting Social Security benefits.[39]

Even after the ADEA banned retirement at age 65, most workers (51% of workers aged 40–69) still faced a mandatory retirement age, usually age 70, according to Labor Department data. Other studies report similar figures, that mandatory retirement covered 40–50 percent of male figures.[40]

Barker and Clark estimated the effect of mandatory retirement on labor-force participation using data from the Social Security Administration's Retirement History Study, which was a ten-year longitudinal national study. Many workers retired voluntarily, either early or at normal ages, or could not continue work because of ill health. About 13 percent of the cohort retired at the mandatory retirement age. Roughly three out of five of the mandatorily retired workers desired to keep working and also were physically able to continue working but were forced to retire. Mandatory retirement thus removed from the labor force about one in twenty of the cohort at age 65.[41] Some other estimates using different methodology reached somewhat higher figures.[42] Two different estimates of what happened to the cohort of male workers approaching age 65 are shown in Figures 2.1 and 2.2.

Nonhiring

In the United States, the over-45 group make up 76 percent of the long-term unemployed.[43] Daniel found that British workers over age 55 were three times more likely to have been made redundant than were workers below age 25.[44] According to a commentary in the *Times,* "age discrimination is widespread" in Britain. In job advertisements, for example, age is frequently the first qualification listed, above experience or achievements. Studies of job vacancies listed with British Government agencies in the late 1970s found that only a quarter were open to those over 50. Among a small number of employers who were surveyed in England, none suggested that age reduces intellec-

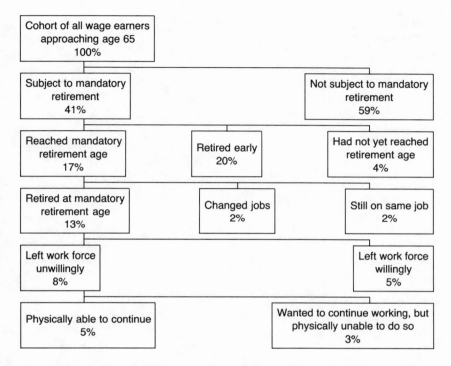

FIGURE 2.1   Incidence of Mandatory Retirement According to the Retirement History Study (1969–73)

Source: Adapted from David T. Barker and Robert L. Clark, "Mandatory Retirement and Labor Force Participation of Respondents in the Retirement History Study," *Social Security Bulletin* 43 (November 1980): 21, 24, and 25.

tual capacity, but they believed older people had less flexibility, motivation, and drive; were unsuited for training, new technology, or new fields of work; and would not fit in with younger workers. Some firms assumed a typical career line and made no allowances for late starters or career breaks. Some used age as a simple means of reducing the otherwise large number of applicants.

The Allocation of Mandatory Retirement

We have information on the allocation by industry and occupation of mandatory retirement practices before its federal regulation. Before the ADEA was adopted in 1967, mandatory retirement was most prevalent in public administration, transportation and public utilities, and manufacturing. The occupa-

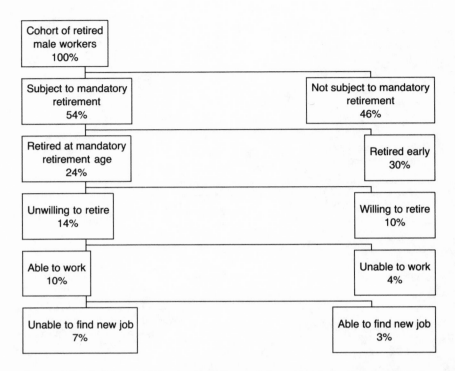

FIGURE 2.2   Incidence of Mandatory Retirement According to the Survey of Newly Entitled Beneficiaries (January–December 1968)

Source: Adapted from James H. Schulz, "The Economics of Mandatory Retirement," *Industrial Gerontology* 1 (Winter 1974): 5, from data appearing in Virginia Reno, "Why Men Stop Working at or before Age 65: Findings from the Survey of New Beneficiaries," *Social Security Bulletin* 34 (June 1971): 3–14.

tions it affected most were teachers, professional or technical workers, and clericals, with substantial impact on all other occupational groups except sales, farm workers, and private household workers.[45]

Other data concern 1969, when slightly less than half (44%) of workers aged 58–61 were in jobs with mandatory retirement rules. The use of age-work rules varied widely. At one extreme, four out of five workers were subject to age-work rules in some industries—communications, transportation, petroleum refineries, instruments, and the federal government. At the other end of the spectrum were industries where only one out of five workers were covered—service industries, sales, and apparel. Among government workers,

86 percent of federal workers were subject to mandatory retirement, 77 percent of state workers, and only 59 percent of local government workers.[46]

The use of mandatory retirement in industries was highly correlated with the extent of pension coverage, a relationship which is consistent with several different explanations of mandatory retirement.

Mandatory retirement rules were more likely in higher-wage industries with white-collar workers. Mandatory retirement was more common for white-collar workers than blue-collar, but more common for highly skilled blue-collar than for low-skilled white-collar. "In addition," the Department of Labor found, "those industries in which physical demand requirements are important tended not to have mandatory retirement rules. . . . Mandatory retirement was more prevalent in occupations that are not physically demanding than in those with rigorous physical requirements."[47] The data on the performance of older workers presented in Part 3 of this book indicates that among workers in their sixties degradation in strength and speed is more likely than is decline in intellectual abilities. The data on the actual incidence of mandatory retirement thus is inconsistent with any simple substantive rationality explanation that such rules are based on decline in worker productivity.

It was usually large firms that had mandatory retirement policies. According to a 1981 study of 1,600 firms by Portland State University, among large firms (500 or more employees) 60 percent had mandatory retirement; among small firms (20–49 employees) only 7 percent did. Similar results were obtained in a 1984 survey of 363 firms conducted by the Conference Board. Among the largest firms (25,000 or more employees) 79 percent had mandatory retirement, although many other large companies had rescinded such policies entirely.[48]

Top executives and tenured professors were covered by special clauses in the ADEA permitting forced retirement at age 65. There was uneven use of that permission: 85 percent of top executives in large firms were subject to such rules, compared to 51 percent of workers generally before the 1986 amendments; one-third of all college professors reaching age 65 in 1981 faced mandatory retirement at that age.[49]

The Costs of Mandatory Retirement

Mandatory retirement entails many personal and social costs as well as benefits.[50] According to Congressman Claude Pepper, "older workers are caught in the jaws of a vise, in which mandatory retirement policies, work disincentives in pension plans and pressure to get out of the workforce early exert force in one direction, while inflation and threatened retirement benefit reductions exert pressure in the other." [51]

Retirement itself, if the replacement ratio is adequate, can be a gift of leisure or an opportunity to do personally valued tasks. Even the mandatory feature of retirement is often praised as facilitating personal and institutional planning and reducing psychic pain for both the older worker and management. But compelled retirement forces people out of their most valued and highly regarded roles, lowering their social status and morale. [52] Job income is terminated and comparable other work is generally not available to the retired person. [53] Pensions and public income sources often provide an insufficient replacement ratio. Earlier research concluded that many retirees received less than half their preretirement income; Palmore and associates found that the average retiree retains about three-fourths of preretirement income. [54] The retired aged have been said to be the social group most vulnerable to inflation, except when benefits and pensions are adequately indexed. [55] Congress tied Social Security benefits to the Consumer Price Index beginning in 1974, but most private pensions are still not indexed; over a recent decade, inflation reduced the purchasing power of private pensions by more than 50 percent. [56] Moreover, the aged, whether working or not, are exposed to the financial drain of catastrophic and long-term illness; the cushion of government health programs for the elderly may be better or may be worse than that provided to working people through job-related health insurance programs. Because financial provisions often are not adequate, many retired elderly find themselves below the poverty level, including many who were not poor during their working lives. [57] Holden and associates found that 30 percent of the couples who were not poor just prior to retirement become poor within the ten years after retirement. [58] During 1987, the Reagan administration and congressional leaders started moving toward enhanced federal benefit programs to cover more of the costs of catastrophic illness for the elderly. [59]

Retirement has different meanings to different people. The 1985 book by Palmore and associates, *Retirement,* and other studies have differentiated the consequences of retirement, depending in part on class, sex, race, and the adequacy of income. Older workers differ among themselves also as to their health and savings, how much they like their jobs, whether or not they are married and the health and work status of the spouse, and the presence of adult children or of their own elderly parents. Women on pensions receive less money than men: median private-pension income for older women is $1,520, compared to $2,980 for men. And fewer women than men receive private pensions: 10 percent of older women do, compared to 29 percent of older men. Minorities fare even worse: 3 percent of black unmarried older women and 12 percent of black unmarried older men receive a private pension. Women and minorities are less likely than white men to retire with adequate private pensions because their employment patterns differ from the type most pension plans reward: long-term, well-paid, full-time, steady employment. In part for these reasons, older women are poorer than older men: women constitute 59 percent of the population over 65, but constitute 71 percent of the aged poor.[60] Congress recognized the obstacles women face in obtaining pension income by passing the Retirement Equity Act that took effect in 1985; this legislation makes it easier for working women to qualify for pensions and protects the rights of wives of working men.[61]

The amount of harm done a worker by forced retirement is relevant to the normative analysis. We would be less likely to regard mandatory retirement as age discrimination if every retired person were to receive full salary: such retirement could conceivably be determined not to be a harm at all, and then the question of its justification would not arise. Of course, if the existence of a pension makes retirement fully voluntary, the question of mandatory retirement hardly arises. In addition to the replacement ratio of pension to prior earnings, the existence of other firms willing to hire the elderly helps determine whether workers suffer severe economic loss at retirement.

But mandatory retirement, even if well paid, is nonetheless open to criticism as arbitrary. By analogy, if an agency head were to relieve women employees of all duties, based on the generalization that women were unfit to do the work, we would raise the question of discrimination even if they still drew full pay. We would want to know whether or not the generalization was accurate, not just how much harm it caused the women. If mandatory retirement is based on false stereotypes, it can be deemed discrimination even if the existence of pensions makes it more palatable.

While mandatory retirement manifests the choice of the employer and sometimes that of a union-employer collective bargaining agreement, it infringes on the decision-making autonomy of the individual employee in a crucial area of his life. It cuts into what many people (and many courts) have long spoken of as a basic right, the right to earn one's living.[62]

Compulsory retirement, with its cessation of productive work, may also be harmful to the mental and physical health of the individual.[63] Congressional debate has referred to gerontological testimony that older unemployed workers experience feelings of uselessness, isolation, and loneliness and have poorer health than those still employed.[64] An often-cited report of the American Medical Association's Committee on Aging even claimed it may lead to premature death, though Robert Atchley's analysis concluded that this is not the case.[65] Earlier studies had concluded that retirees are substantially poorer, sicker, less active, and less satisfied than workers. Palmore and associates differ, at least for voluntary retirees at the normal age, and conclude that while some retirees have health declines, others have health improvements, so that the average retiree has little or no adverse health impact.[66] Ekerdt and associates compared the health of retired persons and a control group of nonretirees. In a detailed study based on medical examinations, they found that the health of those who retire did not deteriorate any more than that of the nonretired.[67]

The Department of Labor identified several reasons for concern about mandatory retirement and the continuing decline in labor-force participation by older persons. The future economic position of an older person may be endangered by early labor force withdrawal since longer periods of retirement are now anticipated under conditions of sustained inflation. It appears that older persons' preferences for part-time employment are increasing but that labor demand is not sufficient to satisfy their current employment needs. Earlier retirements also increase the financial stress on both Social Security and private pension plans. Moreover, shortages of skilled labor could develop in certain industries, as could general labor shortages. For these reasons, the potential for reversing the decline in labor-force participation, and for raising or eliminating the mandatory retirement age, became major public issues.[68]

Moreover, while retirement may appear to be a cost saving to the employer, it imposes a cost on the economy as a whole: in 1977 James Schulz estimated that mandatory retirement of willing and able employees cost the United States $4.5 billion of gross national product.[69] It is unclear what cost retirement imposes on the economy in nations with markedly different conditions.

Alternative Age-Work Practices

The observed characteristics of the mandatory retirement system may be highlighted by contrasting them to possible alternatives.

When forced retirement is based on the supposed diminished competency of the older workers, rational economic behavior by firms would lead to alternative age-work policies (which would not necessarily be as age-neutral as the model of the Age Discrimination in Employment Act). For most firms, it would be desirable for the worker and rational for the employer to have available a variety of flexible options for older workers, such as phased retirement. Such options would enhance individual autonomy and should generally prove profitable for the firm.

For firms that chose to do so it would also be efficient to evaluate individually the productivity of employees who continue past the "usual" retirement age (though the ADEA and seniority systems prohibit limiting such evaluations to the oldest and most senior workers). Fair and accepted evaluation procedures could lead firms and older workers to agree that some older employees were to continue on as usual, other employees were to be involuntarily retired, and still other employees could continue working on renegotiated terms and conditions of employment—such as a switch to another position, partial retirement, or even reverse seniority or lowered wage.

For firms where a nonmonitored atmosphere is preferred, it could sometimes be rational to use age-based generalizations instead of individualized determinations of productivity, if those generalizations were actually based on facts showing that workers of a given age were less likely to perform satisfactorily at a given job. Such age-based generations can only be prima facie valid, however. Rationality requires as a minimum that individuals be allowed to establish that on the actual facts they are exceptions. Where individuals are willing to take on the psychological and financial costs of individualized determination or where, as is common, firms are already making such individualized evaluations of workers, it is not rational to use instead an age-based generalization.

When forced retirement is based on the supposed need to create promotional opportunities, rational economic behavior by institutions would also lead to alternative policies that retain valued older workers.

Flexible Retirement

In the United States, few options short of total retirement are generally available; part-time phased retirement is rarely offered.[70] Phased retirement and other alternative work programs for older workers were recommended at the North American technical meetings for the 1982 U.N. World Assembly on Aging.[71]

A recent poll concluded that most of those now working would like the option, at normal retirement age, to work part-time instead of retiring completely.[72] The results were consistent across age groups (younger adults wanted that option, 75%–18%, those in preretirement years, 79%–18%, and those over 65 and still working, 73%–21%).[73] Among the self-employed elderly (ages 60–64), who are far more likely to control their own work arrangement, part-time work is already 2 1/2 times more common than among salaried or wage employees.[74] And there are other indications that some workers would in fact prefer continued work with adjustment of wages and job assignment rather than retirement.[75] A 1981 Harris poll found that four out of five of workers aged 55–64 said they wanted to combine part-time work with retirement.[76] A field survey of personnel managers concluded that if flexible retirement options existed, management-level workers would often be retained instead of terminated. A related finding is that between a quarter and a third of retired men and women do return to work, according to Palmore and associates. Of the working retired men, nearly half work all year, and almost as many work full-time. Most working retired have a job with the same status as their preretirement job, but there are more downward status shifts than upward ones.[77]

Flexible retirement appears to be a viable alternative to mandatory retirement.[78] Positive employer experience with part-time work for the elderly is reported by Copperman and Keast in *Adjusting to an Older Work Force*. They present as models for change over a dozen innovative employer policies successfully used by various firms.[79] They conclude that flexible employer policies will enable an organization to retain the skills of its older workers while providing promotional opportunities for other workers.[80] Such policies involve part-time work opportunities to satisfy the preferences of older workers for increased leisure time. Other case examples are collected in the computerized files of the National Older Workers Information System (NOWIS).[81] Strategies and initiatives for such programs are also discussed in a report of the National Commission for Employment Policy, an independent federal agency that advises the president and Congress on national employment and training issues.[82]

A firm can build flexibility into the structure of its jobs by beginning early to consider alternative career plans for employees, retraining obsolescent workers, developing plans for lateral transfers, instituting part-time work or phased retirement programs, and considering job-modification programs. The Committee for Economic Development saw the goal as fostering a smoother transition from regular work to retirement, noting such options as voluntary downgrading; greater flexibility in work scheduling and assignment; job sharing, reduced work week, or permanent part-time work; leaves, sabbaticals, or longer vacations; and assignment to community projects.[83] Morrison's study of ways to maximize employment opportunities for the older worker listed similar alternatives.[84]

Part-time work for older employees is encouraged in some countries. In recent years, many industrial countries have modified their social security systems to give older workers more flexibility.[85] Scandinavian countries have used partial pension plans to encourage phased-in retirements; the Swedish plan, adopted in the 1970s, is for partial retirement before normal retirement age, and the Norwegian plan, also from the '70s, encourages partial retirement after the normal retirement age. Since 1976, Swedish workers age 60–64 have been able to opt to reduce their working hours, at a loss of pay, and receive a partial pension. Full old-age benefits are available at age 65, without the necessity of retirement and with no actuarial reduction for prior partial retirement. The Swedish system was proposed by unions; employers preferred collective bargaining on the plan to its adoption by legislation. The purposes of the system are to increase flexibility and freedom of choice about retirement, to provide for a smoother transition from work to retirement, and to ease working conditions during the last years of work.[86] The partial pension replaces up to 50 percent of the lost wages; after taxes, many workers receive 80–85 percent of their prior net earnings. From 21 to 27 percent of those eligible for partial pensions have taken them, according to the Swedish National Social Insurance Board.[87] In Norway, a worker at the normal retirement age of 67 may choose from one-quarter to three-quarters of his or her pension and continue to work part time, so long as the combined income is less than 80 percent of former earnings.

The USSR allows workers to continue working while drawing a pension as an inducement to continue in the work force. Pensioners may be kept on the job either in a part-time capacity or fully employed. This policy is intended to provide a reserve in case of labor shortages, to keep the economy active, and to benefit the mental and physical health and morale of the pensioners.[88] Reports differ on whether allowing Soviet pensioners to continue work has succeeded in inducing them to stay in the labor force.

Period-Specific Retirement Policies

A large number of corporations have tried "exit-incentive" programs, providing for voluntary separation or optional early retirement. A 1986 survey by Hewitt Associates found that about one-third of American corporations surveyed had used such programs in the past five years, generally larger companies with over 50,000 employees. Similarly, a 1984 survey by the Conference Board found that 36 percent of the 363 corporations surveyed had offered such programs at least once since 1970.[89] Seventy-five percent of such programs, according to the Hewitt survey, feature "windows" for early retirement—specific periods within which the eligible employees must decide whether or not to exercise the option to retire. Thus, these retirement programs are period-specific rather than age-specific, apparently based on the needs of their companies at those times, rather than primarily upon assumptions about the qualifications of employees of such ages in general. An example is the retirement policy adopted in 1986 by the Abbey National, Britain's second largest building society. It had recruited large numbers of management trainees in the late 1960s and early 1970s, and therefore by 1986 it had a bulge of junior and middle managers in their late thirties and early forties, and wanted to promote more of them. It also wanted to prepare for major changes in British legal regulation that would alter the nature of its work. The firm inaugurated an early retirement plan for branch managers and other middle managers over 50: they were sent letters inviting them to discuss terms with a personnel counselor if they wanted to retire before the normal age of 60. Those who chose early retirement received a cash bonus and in some cases slightly earlier pension eligibility. In the first two months of the plan, 100 managers were contacted, and "a few" had taken up the offer. A spokesman for the company said there was "no question of the society attempting to get rid" of the over fifties. It is notable that the retirement policy was adjusted to meet a specific cohort and period effect, rather than being based inflexibly on any universal assumption about a certain age group. Moreover, the policy was based on personal choice, offering inducements and counseling, rather than a mandatory rule.[90]

3 • Puzzles and Models

Puzzles of Age-Work Policy

The proposed explanations of age-work practices may all be tested against the actual phenomena, which may be called the puzzles of age-work policy. The phenomena most useful for policy analysis are those that existed when age-work practices were in full bloom, before the substantial inroads on forced retirement at age 65 made by the Age Discrimination in Employment Act Amendments of 1978. Twelve puzzles, each of them characteristic of modern American age-work practices, may be identified:

1. A relationship (the *age-work effect*) exists between chronological old age and lowered participation in the work force. A key component of the relationship is involuntary—an exclusion from the work force by age-based policies of mandatory retirement and nonhiring.
2. These mandatory retirement policies are based on chronological age rather than on a more complete assessment of individual characteristics. Generalization substitutes for individualized assessment. Assuming that age per se is not the functional characteristic upon which retirement is premised but is a proxy for that characteristic, then mandatory retirement policies involve generalizations that aged workers share an actual functional characteristic (e.g., unsatisfactory job performance or productivity/wage ratio).
3. The mandatory retirement policies adopt some *specific* age at which retirement is required.
4. Mandatory retirement policies generally do not allow workers to negotiate to permit continued employment past the usual retirement age, in different capacities or at different wages. The employment decision process is binary rather than continuous.
5. Furthermore, many firms adopt *automatic* mandatory retirement policies that withdraw from management the discretion to continue individual employees past the fixed retirement age. The last-mentioned characteristic is something like self-paternalism, Odysseus having himself tied to the mast so he would not be able later to do what he would then want.
6. Employers also adopt bars against new hiring of the elderly similar to the mandatory retirement policies.

37

7. According to some data, unions sometimes bargain for mandatory retirement plans even when no private pension benefits are provided in the negotiated contract.
8. In addition, according to some data, older persons in general or older union members, more than younger ones or nonmembers, support retirement plans.
9. Larger firms are more likely than smaller ones to have mandatory retirement policies.
10. Firms with pension plans are more likely than others to have mandatory retirement policies.
11. Nevertheless, firms of the same size and type, at the same time, may differ in their age-work policies.
12. Mandatory retirement practices show an inverted U trend over time. They were first instituted on a large scale in the late nineteenth and early twentieth centuries, were increasingly accepted particularly after World War II, but in recent years have declined in acceptance in the United States.

Further empirical research, or meta-analysis[1] of prior studies may clarify, extend, and quantify this list of characteristics.

A Typology of Causal Theories

Possible causes of mandatory retirement will be set out briefly, grouped into four types of models.

In brief, *rationality* explanations state that age-work policies are economically rational. Several explanations argue that the employer adopts a specific age-work policy for the purpose of maximizing profits (or the equivalent achievement of goals for a governmental or nonprofit agency). Such explanations may stress that the policy is *substantively rational* (aged workers are not cost-effective, e.g., because they are likely to be less productive), or that it has *systemic* value (e.g., fresh blood is needed or promotional opportunities must be created), or that it achieves *process rationality* (e.g., by reducing the costs of making individualized determinations).[2] Process rationality explanations overlap explanations in terms of the psychology of the personnel process and a preference for routinization.

Another group of explanations emphasize the *macroeconomic* context in which employer decisions are made, such as changes in the size of the available labor pool or the need for enhanced national productivity. For such explanations to be persuasive, the macroeconomic context must be related to individual choices of private employers, as rationality explanations directly provide. Some macroeconomic explanations look to marketplace interactions between the elderly and younger workers: intergroup competition may be a process in which younger workers as a group compete with a group of older workers for scarce jobs. Some of these explanations see the older workers as primarily in competition with women or minority groups; age-work practices are then thought to reflect the success of the groups in the competition. In a variant version, union policy rather than the labor marketplace is identified as the locus where intergroup rivalries are expressed. How such competition influences employer practices must be explained here also: perhaps unions seek mandatory retirement rules in their collective bargaining.

A third set of explanations focuses on the individual worker's *intertemporal choices,* which allocate work and leisure over a life cycle and thus determine some particular retirement age. Employer age-work practices are thought to mimic these individual choices. The mechanism by which employer practices are influenced must still be explicated: presumably common worker preferences determine what workers or their unions bargain for, as well as what generalizations about workers' behavior employers will make. Alternatively, employers are thought to impose an age-earnings profile associated with long-term contracting and mandatory retirement.

A final set of *attitudinal* explanations look to culture and to psychology. Intergenerational attitudes may be emphasized. Under these explanations, employers are thought to adopt age-work policies because of attitudes towards the elderly, based on psychological or cultural causes such as factual stereotyping, emotional prejudice, or unconscious ambivalence. Prejudiced personnel practices may reflect attitudes of the employer, other workers, or customers. Prejudiced behavior is sometimes analyzed as equivalent to a "taste for discrimination."[3]

Other cultural changes and psychological processes that have been proposed as salient involve labor-management attitudes rather than intergenerational attitudes. Routinization of decisions in large, bureaucratic firms could be a general trend subsuming the specific practices on retirement. There may also be a psychology of the personnel process such that managers or workers have a distaste for evaluation of workers. If there is a specific unease with evaluating older workers, the explanation would overlap both intergenerational attitudes and process rationality. Under this set of explanations, age-work policies may maximize the private (emotional or even neurotic) utilities of management officials who make personnel decisions, while not necessarily maximizing the firm's profits.

These models may be compared with the views of economically rational behavior employed by some of the scholars writing in the movement known as

Law and Economics.[4] Many of the models can be viewed as fitting within the assumption that social patterns reflect rational economic maximization. The model which was denominated "rational" posits that the age-work effect is produced by profit-maximizing behavior on the part of employers. The macroeconomic explanations assume overall rationality, though not always spelling out the connection between broad context and the behavior of individual firms. The rivalry form of the model assumes that the age-work effect is produced by competitive pressures among groups of younger and older workers, that may, for example, be effectuated through collective bargaining agreements establishing retirement plans.[5] The intertemporal choice model can be viewed as tracing the age-work effect to the maximization of the career-long preferences of the worker, preferences which would be reflected in the employment patterns offered by the market, or depend on the firm's attempt to manipulate the age-earnings profile to maximize profits.[6] The psychological and cultural models, however, assume that the age-work effect does not maximize external, real-world monetary satisfactions. In one version of this model, the practice is assumed to occur because it maximizes unconscious psychic satisfactions. In terms of Freud's differentiation, the age-work effect then would not serve the reality principle by rationally maximizing satisfaction over the long run but, rather, occurs because it serves the pleasure principle, maximizing immediate satisfaction of needs which are often unconscious and symbolic, and may even be self-defeating.[7]

Making use of this typology of causes of age-work practices, Parts 2 and 3 review the empirical and theoretical research studies in the literature on the subject. In Part 4 the models will be explicated in more detail, providing an overview of the research; empirical conclusions are set out; and the normative implications of the study will be suggested.

II • The Studies of Mandatory Retirement

Issues of age-work policy were discussed in Part 1; research data and theoretical analyses relevant to the issues are analyzed in this and the next part. Part 2 reviews studies bearing directly on explanations of mandatory retirement. Part 3 deals with extrinsic assumptions about aging, the older worker, and ageism that are involved in some of the explanations.

Since there is no existing review of this body of literature, this summary of the studies should have value to those concerned with these issues. And since the work of others is the data for my reasoning, it is a matter of fairness that their research be set out independently.

The studies cited do not fit neatly in the typology of models which I set out in Part 1: many of the authors present analyses consistent with more than one of the alternative explanations. Each study is nevertheless largely discussed in one place, as it would be confusing to split the discussion. Some require major detours to justify acceptance or rejection of them.

An integrated statement of the conclusions drawn from this body of research and my own analyses are set out in Part 4.

4 • Discrimination and Stereotype Theories

A group of studies from the late 1930s through the 1950s invoked both discrimination and substantive rationality as explanations of mandatory retirement.

Early Use of the Discrimination Concept

One of the earliest explanations of age-work practices was set out in a brief article "Causes of Discrimination against Older Workers" published in 1938, summarizing the report of a New York State legislative committee and drawing on two earlier surveys.[1] The report is concerned with nonhiring, rather than with mandatory retirement (as indeed was the original version of the ADEA),[2] and in this context its discussion of the "older worker" meant the middle-aged worker. There was at that time little developed law about a constitutional right against any form of discrimination; the committee's report dealt with discrimination against older workers not from the point of view of constitutional or natural rights, but as a social problem to be dealt with by legislation. To this end it attempted a "complete and thorough inquiry."

The New York State committee found that nonhiring could create enforced poverty; moreover, when "one is denied employment while still in full possession of one's physical and mental facilities it must indeed be discouraging." Discrimination in hiring middle-aged workers was found to exist in practically all industrial areas of New York State. Nevertheless, "manufacturers, especially the large employers, have not cared to admit any discrimination in the hiring of older workers," according to the committee.[3] The statement suggests that "discrimination" was meant in a pejorative sense and that the practice, even if believed to be rational, was regarded as unpopular or embarrassing.

The "alleged causes of discrimination" against hiring the middle-aged were surveyed by the committee by hearing testimony from employers, unions, and others representing almost a third of New York workers. Most reasons given in the testimony were substantively rational. A first group related to age-related decline: middle-aged workers were believed less efficient, less trainable, more susceptible to occupational disease, often physically unfit because of industrial accidents, and subject to a higher accident rate. A second group of reasons related to modernization: there was a speed-up in industry; old skills had become obsolete; old jobs had been destroyed by modern machinery, new methods, or the decline of old industries. An additional reason was based on age per se (or at least older appearance): the public was said to demand younger workers for some jobs, like waitress or salesclerk.

A substantively rational cohort effect was also noted. Middle-aged workers often could not write legibly or figure accurately; they often lacked high-school or trade-school training; many had lost skills during layoffs in the Depression. Another reason, not based on decline in productivity but on productivity-wages ratio, was that the young could be hired more cheaply. A further set of reasons, related to insurance, seems to be derivative of beliefs about older workers. Workmen's compensation insurance rates would rise; group insurance rates would rise; insurance companies urged hiring the young. Similarly, there would be increased rates for employers under their own pension plans.

Finally, the committee noted, without ascribing any reason, the existence of "discrimination" against the middle-aged in government civil service rules.

The committee found that some of these beliefs about older workers were factual. It agreed that medicine had established that among wage earners, though perhaps not "higher social groups," there was a marked "degeneration" after age 40. The committee's words on this point are worthy of quotation as evidencing enlightened opinion half a century ago: "Medical authorities are agreed that from the fortieth year, there is a marked physiological degeneration which becomes accelerated with the passage of time and which ends with death. When the process of physiological involution does set in, the degeneration is speeded up greatly, is more widespread, and many more impairments become evidenced in a shorter period of time among wage earners than among higher social groups."[4]

Some employer beliefs were found by the committee not to be factual; for example, workmen's compensation rates did not rise. Still other beliefs were accurate in part but, the committee implied, not sufficient basis for across-the-board policies. For example, a few insurance companies did urge hiring the young; though older workers took longer to recuperate, they were in fact less liable to accidents; while many had had industrial accidents, an "amazingly high rate" were nevertheless employable; and skilled older workers were not so susceptible to occupational disease. In general, with employer effort, many of the perceived problems could be overcome.

The impression one gains from the report is that most of the causes for not hiring older workers derived from beliefs as to age-related degeneration. The committee seemed to think that many of these beliefs did have some basis. Nevertheless, it concluded that they were not sufficient to justify the hiring practices, which as a whole were condemnable as "discrimination."

Other Early Surveys of Firms

In the post–World War II period, additional studies continued to explain mandatory retirement in terms of discrimination and substantive rationality.

In 1951, Fox surveyed 168 Minneapolis firms on mandatory retirement. He found that, among firms without pension plans, 45 percent reported that *all* employees reaching 65 could still handle their usual jobs. Some added that employees who would have had difficulty handling their usual jobs after 65 had either been discharged or put on jobs which they could handle before they reached 65.[5] Thus, a significant number of firms found neither a substantive nor process-rationality basis for a mandatory retirement rule: most workers remained able, and those that did not could be identified feasibly.

Fox's general conclusion was that the firms which had compulsory-retirement pension plans were the ones that let all workers go at 65. Firms without such a plan continued most or all workers except for the few who voluntarily retired. Of nonpension firms, 93 percent kept on "most or all" hourly employees, and 87 percent kept "most or all" salaried employees, after age 65.

He thus found that a large proportion of firms—those with pensions—implemented retirement practices which resulted in the loss of workers who could still handle their usual jobs satisfactorily. By contrast, one half of the firms without pension plans said that "most or all" hourly employees who could *not* handle their usual jobs were nevertheless kept on after 65; only one firm with a pension plan said this.

Fox wondered why most firms with pension plans enforced a compulsory retirement policy when it meant losing good employees whose work was recognized as satisfactory by management. The answers he received in interviews closely paralleled those reported in other studies, such as that of Brower in 1944.[6] Some of the reasons emphasized substantive rationality. It was not so much that the workers at 65 had been found to be less productive but that some managers feared that such employees are liable to sudden deterioration in the near future. (Fox pointed out that the limited research data then available did not indicate that age 65 has any special significance, but suggested that old age makes itself felt beginning at about 70.)[7] No process rationality reasons were given, in the sense that individualized determinations were difficult or expensive to make; Fox did not note significant costs (psychic or otherwise) of screening out those not qualified. Systemic rationality reasons were given: many managers believed that unless older people were retired, promotion channels for younger workers were clogged. Research showed that younger workers look forward to promotions, while older workers had little expectation of better jobs.[8] This explanation was not, however, generally applicable: many senior manual workers were at the top of their craft and did not want promotions into supervisory positions.

Intergenerational attitudes were mentioned, not in the sense that management did not like older workers, but in the sense that they believed that younger and older workers do not work well together. Indeed, limited research data suggested that foremen have even less favorable attitudes to older people than do employees in general. Yet these reasons would not have necessitated a retirement policy; Fox cited a British study suggesting using separate work groups for older workers as an alternative way to deal with the problems. As for nonhiring of the older worker, Fox cited surveys from 1929, 1938, and 1949 as giving practically identical reasons: fear that group insurance premiums would increase and the belief that older workers have more accidents. Qualifying clauses in pension plans were also mentioned in several surveys. Fox found little documentation to support these management worries; for example, he reported extensive research showing that older workers have fewer accidents, though more severe ones.[9]

A routinization reason given was that individualized determinations were difficult to justify to unions. For example, one firm previously had tried to retain after 65 those employees who could still handle their usual jobs, but workers not retained filed grievances. Rather than face the handling of grievances, the firm switched to retiring all employees at age 65.

Fox concluded that an automatic retirement policy was not justified; a large proportion of older people are able to compete on equal terms with younger workers, and the use of training programs, job adaptation, and transfers can enhance the utilization of older workers. Fox therefore regarded age-work retirement policies as an attribute of traditional pension plans not explicable by economic rationality.

Another study of firms with pension plans, by Brower in 1944, complements that of Fox by giving some evidence as to how the age for retirement was fixed. Two-thirds of all plans then set the age at 65, "which coincides with the age fixed under the Social Security Act."[10] Before federal old-age benefits became effective, it was a widespread practice to retire women many years earlier. Under the new law the tendency was to set the date at 65 for both sexes. Thus, major changes in retirement practice were made without benefit of any new data on productivity or health.[11]

Worthy of note is testimony from a Massachusetts statistician that in a state survey on older workers a "large number" of firms explicitly reported that they used no maximum hiring-age limit, but that further investigation showed that many of them actually did have such limits, "often without realizing it." [12] This testimony suggests that age-work practices were not always imposed from the top in large bureaucracies, as is sometimes hypothesized, but often grew out of the practices of those who did the hiring.

5 • Macroeconomic Theories

Several studies emphasize the importance of macroeconomic factors in causing age-work practices.

Displacement

The economic historian Clarence Long considered age-work issues in a chapter of his 1958 book, *The Labor Force under Changing Income and Employment.*[1] Long's method was to compare quantitative data from various periods. His study considered the wider topic of labor force participation by older workers, but nevertheless sheds light on mandatory retirement policies. He found that during the first half of this century men over 45 reduced their participation in the labor force sizeably, and men over 65 far more.

Long concluded that the circumstantial evidence suggested that older men were to a large extent displaced by the entrance into the labor force of better-trained women, available at lower wages. He rejected several alternative causal explanations. His conclusions were that the decline has not been closely related to the level of unemployment, nor to the rise in real income (at least since 1930), nor to the extension of pensions and of Social Security (at least before 1940), nor to any discoverable deterioration in average physical ability to work (compared with men of the same age in earlier decades), nor to changes in self-employment opportunities or rapidity of technological change. Over the long run, also, Long found participation by older men lower in some recent high-employment years than in earlier years of considerable unemployment.[2]

Specifically addressing the question of why age-work policies exist, Long considered several factors. Substantively rational reasons were given by some employers, who asserted productivity explanations for age-work policies.[3] Age-work policies often exist in chain stores, hotels, and restaurants, where the younger workers are considered more attractive to customers—a substantively rational reason, but one applying only to those industries. (This industry-specific explanation is consistent with MacDonald's views.)[4] Long also considered but rejected the hypothesis that technological advancement renders the elderly less efficient.[5] Rapid technological changes had led to the observation that "half of education is out-of-date in ten years"[6] and that productivity drops off in the mid-thirties when "obsolescence" sets in. (The theory of technological obsolescence appears still to be applied to both managers and employees in modern high-technology fields such as aerospace engineering, but seems to have less to do with old age retirement.)[7]

In his book Long put forward a version of what we may call the "age-bonus" thesis, later advanced by Lazear,[8] which Long thought particularly important with white-collar workers. He called attention to the practice of giving automatic raises, frequently on the basis of years of service, without close attention to efficiency; the practice was presumably justified on process rationality grounds. He argued that older workers may gradually reach wage levels above their productivity; they consequently will be replaced by younger and lower-paid workers whenever a good excuse presents itself.

A systemically rational reason noted by Long was that some employers had a policy of keeping promotion channels clear to keep ambitious young people from leaving.[9] Similarly, age-work rules are associated with policies of hiring only at the bottom and promoting from within.

A process rationality explanation was also considered.[10] With rapid industrialization and the growth of large corporations, it became more difficult to make individual determinations, and industry tried to standardize its personnel policies to apply to large numbers of employees. Compulsory retirement at an arbitrary age then became the easiest way out. The process rationality reason based on firm size received some confirmation from a survey of major industry groups in seven labor markets areas.[11] The survey showed a clear tendency for the proportion of workers over 65 to be smaller the larger the number of employees in the establishment. But Long calculated that the average size of firms had not been increasing fast enough to explain the trend of declining participation by older workers in the work force. (It should be noted again that this figure dealt with labor-force participation rates, not just their involuntary component.)

Long was receptive to the hypothesis that reorganizations based on technological changes may lead to older workers' losing seniority or moral claims on the employer.[12] But he did not find support for the proposition that the industries with the most rapid technological change or the greatest growth in industry size have the fewest older employees. Long did not consider the hypothesis that size and technological change lead to impersonality.

Intergroup competition was the reason most appealing to Long: he italicized his conclusion that employers would not have been so ready to part with the elderly as a source of labor supply if there had not been women available to take those workers' places. Women were preferable employees because of their superior education, a substantively rational reason. "The elderly male has indeed fallen far behind in the ability to compete in the labor market if formal schooling is any index."[13] Long discussed this factor without consid-

49

eration of the cohort effect: contrary to his implicit point, there does not exist some single group of elderly who have fallen behind; rather there are successive cohorts, each of which received increasing amounts of education while young. (If one has only longitudinal data for one cohort, one is not able to distinguish the effects of aging from the effects of the specific period through which the individuals had lived.)[14]

Long assumed that employers hesitate to hire at a lower than usual wage rate. Thus, *a fortiori,* he would have believed that firms disfavored the renegotiation of lower wages for continuing employees. The minimum wage also sets a floor below which some worker's productivity may fall, leading to dismissal rather than renegotiation. Long also regarded some workers as so inferior as not to be useful at any wage rate, and suspected that poor education may be used as a proxy characteristic to identify such workers.

Intertemporal choice as an explanation was implicitly rejected by Long, who believed that people want to work as long as they are physically able to do so. (His belief was later contradicted: high rates for voluntary retirement exist now that more adequate pensions are available.) Long found that the labor-force participation rate had not been closely related over substantial time periods to the rise in real incomes or the extension of pensions and social security; this finding supported his conclusion that age-work policies were not a proxy for personal choice by workers to leave the labor market.

Long also considered "arbitrary discrimination" against older workers, an intergenerational attitude. He did not see why such discrimination should exist at all. He concluded that it was not certain that discrimination had increased during the period that labor-force participation of older workers had decreased.

Long's study therefore supports the thesis of intergroup competition for jobs, particularly between older workers and young, educated women. While he considered labor-force participation rather than mandatory retirement, the two subjects converge given his assumption that few workers at that period voluntarily chose to retire.

Labor Surplus

Long's conclusion may be compared to the similar thesis that the most important factor affecting employment of the older worker is general labor supply and demand, and that when jobs are scarce, older workers are retired or not hired.[15]

There is historical support for this thesis in government benefit policy, union practice, and employer personnel practices. It is widely accepted that one of the major considerations in the establishment of old-age benefits in the United States was to draw elderly persons off the labor market and thus help restore the balance of supply and demand for labor.[16] And union policy, though inconsistent at different periods, sometimes sought to negotiate contracts to remove excess labor from a rapidly automating industry.[17]

An explanation in terms of labor surplus can be tested against some of the characteristics of age-work policies listed earlier. If not supplemented, it does not sufficiently explain the basic age-work phenomenon of differential treatment of older employees in job markets, for it does not indicate why the employer singles out the older worker. Moreover, the reasoning does not explain why there have been reforms raising the retirement age at times when unemployment is high.

A study of mandatory retirement by Juanita Kreps, later Secretary of Commerce, reasoned that when there is labor surplus, the bidding for limited jobs must either force some workers out of jobs or push down the wage rate.[18] There is, however, limited downward flexibility of wages (the *ratchet effect*), and thus higher-paid workers tend to be pushed out. In particular, workers who have pensions available are expected to vacate their jobs in favor of younger men. Kreps's analysis may be compared to that of Long, in terms of intergroup competition. To Kreps the younger are favored for two reasons. First, they have greater financial needs. Though Kreps does not carry the point further, this reasoning seems based on an assumption that younger persons will support families, but older ones will not, an assumption which rests in turn on intergenerational cultural attitudes. Second, the young have better education and up-to-date skills and so presumably are more productive—a substantive rationality explanation.

Kreps's article on labor force participation of the aged also mentions several factors effecting age-work policies. Firms have tended to grow in size, and larger firms have been more likely to adopt age-related policies, for reasons not mentioned but presumably relating to routinization. Second, hiring-age ceilings have become "necessary corollaries" to private pension plans, because "firms are increasingly reluctant to hire workers who have not enough working years left to acquire any significant pension claims."[19] This reluctance appears to be a matter of intergenerational attitude. We might question whether the expression of a company's claimed benevolence in refusal to hire older workers instead suggests unconscious ambivalence. Additional data supporting Kreps's reasoning is now available from international employers: a French firm which did not hire older workers, for example, is quoted as mentioning as a reason "the moral responsibility of taking on a fairly old worker if he has to be dismissed soon afterwards."[20]

Kreps also mentions a systemic rationality factor: compulsory retirement is required to allow promotion from within, thus retaining younger employees and providing incentives for the whole work force.

Finally, she presents several points related to seniority. In theory, "equity" would base promotions on merit, but union-management agreement has substituted reliance on seniority. Seniority involves a "conflict of interest between the young and the older worker" that we call intergroup competition. Kreps suggests that "seniority rules may have contributed significantly to the development of compulsory retirement policies." She believes that seniority systems "in providing some security to workers between, say, 45 and 65, reduced the chances for the 65-year-old retaining his job."[21] Kreps sees this as a matter of "conflict of interest," that is, of intergroup competition. She does not consider whether it also involves intertemporal choice or the psychology of the process.

Prejudices and Labor Supply

The Secretary of Labor's 1965 report, *The Older American Worker: Age Discrimination in Employment,* was accompanied by a volume, *Research Materials,* that included a report by Sara Leiter which was also separately published as "Hiring Policies, Prejudices, and the Older Worker."[22] Leiter's report was based on a special survey conducted by government employment services of firms that hired 89,000 new workers during 1964. The study found that job opportunities for older workers diminish markedly with advancing years after age 45. Over 90 percent of those hired were below 45. Older workers were hired at less than one-third their proportional representation among the unemployed.

About 25 percent of employers imposed upper age limits for one or more occupations; 60 percent of private-sector firms hired older workers in below-average proportions. It was clear to Leiter that labor supply-demand relationships were an important influence on hiring practices, though employers rarely mentioned that reason. Upper age limits tended to vanish, or to be imposed at more advanced ages, for occupations which were hard to fill, both the much-in-demand skilled and professional occupations, and the less-sought-after service and sales jobs. The reasons employers gave for their restrictive policies on hiring older workers "included some related to job performance and others entirely divorced from job performance."[23] Employers emphasized physical capability and also expressed concern with efficiency, productivity, economy, desirable personnel practices, public image, and need for suitable workers.

Other firms had quite a different practice. An affirmative policy of hiring without regard to age was held in one out of six establishments, including retail trades, hotels, personal and medical services, and government. Some of the private firms targeted substantial recruitment efforts at those over 45. Major reasons cited by employers who preferred to hire older workers included older workers' stability, dependability, knowledge, and experience. Other reasons given were less absenteeism, good work habits and attitudes, ability or skills, quality or quantity of work, pride in work, and consistent performance and adaptability.

About 60 percent of establishments made exceptions to their upper age limits. Their explanations as to why they did so "gave convincing proof that labor supply conditions outweighed any considerations which motivated the stipulation of upper age limits."[24] Leiter does not explain why the other 40 percent, which made no exceptions, resisted the forces of supply and demand.

In multiestablishment companies, home offices "often" determined hiring policy relating to age, while in somewhat more than half the firms the policy was determined by officials of the local establishments. Leiter does not point out that this finding undercuts the theory that the need for central control in large bureaucracies encourages age-work policies.

Surveying the reasons given for not hiring older workers, Leiter notes that no employers felt they were acting arbitrarily or capriciously. Nevertheless, she suspected that some were guided by "preconceptions rather than relevant experience."[25] The reason each employer gave often seemed impressive, but the reasons in the aggregate were often inconsistent or contradictory. "In short, it is possible to run the gamut of reasons that employers give for not hiring older persons and then find that other employers hire them because they believe that the exact opposite is true."[26] Some firms, for example, said they did not hire older workers because they lack adaptability; others, just because they are adaptable. Some firms hired older workers for the same jobs from which others excluded them. We should note that although the hiring firms did have experience with older workers, the nonhiring firms may not have had.

Policies of nonhiring sometimes lacked a rational basis. Nonhiring firms sometimes failed to distinguish between jobs which required great physical strength and endurance and those which did not. Their policies were set without any objective standards for determining whether there is some age at which workers could not do a particular job. And their policies made no provision for individual differences, "which are enormous."[27] Additionally, many employers recommended retraining for older workers in up-to-date skills or more marketable jobs but still expressed reluctance to hire them even with such training.

The conclusions implicit in Leiter's study seem to be that macroeconomic factors—the conditions of labor supply and demand—set outer limits to acceptable age-based hiring practices. At least some of the reasons for setting particular age-work policies within that range were based on intergenerational attitudes, "preconceptions rather than relevant experience." She thus recommended "an intensive informational and educational program to encourage employers to consider older applicants for employment strictly on the basis of the individual's ability to perform the job."[28] Leiter did not consider why some firms, though not others, had adopted apparently irrational policies. Nor did she explain why government education programs, rather than market pressures and self-interest, were needed to encourage firms to acquire and make use of such easily available information.

Similar conclusions were reached by Copperman and Keast. They concluded that age has been used as a sorting device by employers for process rationality reasons: age is an easy criterion to use, compared to the high cost of developing individualized methods. Age-based devices, though, are irrational: not only do they terminate unproductive older individuals, but they also undervalue many effective older workers. Continued use of inefficient age-based proxies is possible only in times of labor surplus: "The aggressive recruitment of older workers by employers confronting labor shortages suggests that assumed reductions in productivity related to age are not sufficiently large to influence employers confronting staffing problems; employers' 'tastes for age discrimination' apparently disappear quickly in the face of labor shortages and declining numbers of younger workers."[29]

The Dependency Ratio

There is another macroeconomic explanation of age-work practices aside from that of labor supply and demand. The explanation focuses on the dependency ratio, the ratio of the part of the population which is productively employed to the part which is dependent. It has been suggested, for example, that the postponement of the usual mandatory retirement age from 65 to 70 effected by the ADEA Amendments of 1978 was motivated in part by the need then perceived to keep the Social Security trust fund in balance.[30] Attention to Social Security finances is a manifestation of the requirement that society have an acceptable dependency ratio between employed and nonemployed portions of the population.[31]

Similar reasoning has been used by Graebner to suggest that the previous selection of 65 as the usual mandatory retirement age was influenced by what was an acceptable dependency ratio at that time. Kreps concluded that the distribution of lifetime between working years and leisure years depends primarily on the productivity of labor and hence the extent to which nonworking time can be supported. She contrasted the growth of leisure in the United States—by reducing the labor force at both ends of the worklife span—with a European tendency to lengthen the weekend and the annual vacation.[32] In the United States, during this century the number of nonworking years has grown by about nine years for a male at birth. This nevertheless has amounted to only about one-third the amount of free time added through work week reductions, added vacations, and the like.[33]

An analysis based on the dependency ratio perhaps explains what range of labor-force participation rates by older persons, and what retirement ages, a society could afford. It does not sufficiently explain why employers act as they do to create the observed characteristics of mandatory retirement and other age-work practices. Haber criticizes economic historians who explain these practices in terms of the aggregate work force for not explaining the differences between industries and firms that do and those that do not establish such age-related policies.[34]

Job Rationing

Supplementing the macroeconomic theories is the job-rationing thesis offered by Furstenberg and Thrall.[35] They argue that cultural and normative assumptions create a job-rationing ideology, a system of shared beliefs about who should have preferred access to scarce jobs. These beliefs operate like a queueing mechanism, placing individuals in line for employment. (Phelps had earlier written of "queue unemployment.")[36] The individual's belief about his or her right to a job and obligation to work affect job-seeking behavior. Employers justify hiring practices not only in terms of capability but also in terms of who has the greatest claim to employment—the same kind of fairness argument noted earlier. The aged, along with the young, the handicapped, and women with small children, are often regarded as less entitled to a job.[37] Government policies also embody the job-rationing ideology; for example, the Social Security earnings test penalizes work by individuals between normal retirement age and age 72.

The job-rationing thesis serves to explain the age-work effect: Furstenberg and Thrall's analysis deals explicitly with nonhiring, and we may extend their discussion to mandatory retirement. As a supplement to macroeconomic theories, the cultural queuing mechanism explains how the retirement age is fixed and can account for secular trends in the age fixed: the need for workers dictates how far down the queue employers look. To the extent that the thesis suggests the importance of beliefs about who should work and the relative unimportance of workers' productivity, it explains the age-work phenomena of generalization, absence of renegotiation, and nondiscretionary policies. As a theory about norms, the thesis explains the positions of unions and older workers. The characteristics of age-work policies that remain unexplained by this theory are the existence of variations in policies by size of firm and among similar firms.

Furstenberg and Thrall hint why employers would find the job-rationing ideology in their self-interest: it is systemically rational for them as part of "a grand cover-up of the shortage of jobs," for it "cools out" of the labor force large numbers of people who might otherwise be regarded as unemployed.[38] The retired older worker is just not considered to be unemployed, because she is no longer seeking work. Thus, the ideology reduces social unrest. These authors' explanation is insufficient, however, because they do not explain how it came to be that the elderly were defined as one of the groups occupying places far back in the queue, nor what motivates elderly persons to accept that cultural definition.

The proponents of the several theories discussed in this chapter have presented extensive data and several hypotheses on the causes of age-work practices, all invoking some sort of competition among potential workers for scarce jobs. Under conditions of competition, an alternative result would be that wage rates fall until the market reaches equilibrium. If, however, a ratchet effect keeps the wage rate steady, exclusion of some workers is another means by which the market can reach equilibrium. Age-work policies are a form of such exclusion. All these theories also require some explanation of why older workers lose out in the competition or rationing—either a reason why it is economically rational for employers to prefer young workers, or some attitude of employers not justified on purely economic grounds.

6 • The Age-Bonus Theory

Against the background of this material, let us now turn our attention to Edward Lazear's recent major theory.[1]

Age-Earnings Profile as Incentive

Some economists consider a labor contract similar to a mortgage, with the wage merely an installment payment on a long-term implicit commitment to transfer a certain amount of wealth for a certain amount of labor services.[2] Edward Lazear is one of several authors who have considered, within such a long-term perspective, how the age-earnings profile can be altered to provide incentive effects.[3] His theory of the age-earnings profile yields an explanation of firms' adoption of mandatory retirement.

Lazear's thesis is that firms with mandatory retirement policies also have wage policies that pay younger workers less than their value-marginal product (VMP) and pay older workers more than their VMP. While Lazear does not use the term, one may call the overpayment the *age bonus*.

Lazear does not explicitly specify the form of the age bonus, but it is well known that many firms give annual wage increases without regard to increased productivity, along with noncash compensation in the form of enhanced seniority rights. Lazear presumes that such a wage schedule is regarded by both employers and employees as preferable to a wage schedule equating wages and VMP. Employers prefer the hypothesized schedule because it promotes loyalty and worker diligence, thereby increasing total productivity and enhancing profits. Employees prefer such a schedule because the enhanced profits are shared with them.

Similarly, Hall argued that greater rewards are paid to senior employees so as to motivate younger workers toward hard work and eventual achievement of those rewards.[4] Long's related theory was mentioned in the last section. A thesis similar to Lazear's has also been proposed by Schrank and Waring, who used the term *gap hypothesis*.[5] In this explanation, young people entering a firm are assigned a level beneath their capacities. The pace of improvement in reward is fastest early in the career; later in the career the pace slows, as the gap between contribution and reward is narrowed. There is some research suggesting that as the employee's time in the organization increases, the likelihood of staying with the firm increases while the likelihood of a promotion decreases, consistent with the hypothesis.[6] Schrank and Waring agree with Lazear that the rate of increase in compensation is steeper than the rate of increase in VMP. Unlike Lazear, however, they regard it as rare that the two lines cross to create a "negative gap" justified as compensation for past inequitable treatment. There is little research on promotion past the level of competence.[7] While such promotion (at least as to compensation) is postulated by Lazear to be a regular concomitant of mandatory retirement policy, Schrank and Waring view the phenomenon as a relatively rare instance of the "Peter principle."[8]

Lazear's theory explains mandatory retirement in terms of intertemporal choice. Interestingly, on Lazear's assumptions one need not conclude that the mandatory retirement employer believes that there are age-related declines in productivity, since if there is a practice of age bonuses even an employee with a constant VMP may come to have a wage greater than his VMP.

Lazear assumes that workers and employees either implicitly or explicitly choose a lifetime wage schedule such that the rate of increase in wages exceeds the rate of increase in the VMP of the worker, for the motives stated above. He assumes also that, *ex ante,* the present value of the future wages equals the present value of the future VMP contributed by the worker. These assumptions require that at some time during the course of the worker's employment, his wage will be equal to his VMP at that time, and that at later times his wage will exceed his VMP. These assumptions may appear to require that there be a fixed point in time, *T,* when employment will be mandatorily discontinued. The argument would be that to do otherwise and allow continued employment under the hypothesized conditions would cause the *ex ante* value of the future wages to exceed the *ex ante* value of the worker's contributions to value. If one were to assume that all employees work until death, one could calculate a wage schedule by setting *T* at the actuarial estimate of average death. Under this arrangement, workers who retired early would be paying a high opportunity cost for leisure.

One could imagine an alternative plan, more acceptable to workers, in which *T* is set at the predicted average voluntary retirement date. If *T* were set correctly, the employer would be indifferent because early retirers would balance late retirers. Further, employee choice would be maximized by the voluntary retirement characteristic of the alternative. It is true that, with older workers being paid a wage greater than VMP, they would have an incentive to continue working longer than they "ought" (in productivity terms). It would not be necessary to retain some form of involuntary rationing of these "overpaid" jobs, however, as the average retirement date and the wage schedule could be estimated taking this factor into effect.[9]

Richard Craswell has pointed out that Lazear's theory requires some explanation in terms of information costs or Herbert Simon's concept of "bounded rationality"; otherwise, each older employee's productivity could be assessed on an individual basis.[10] There would be information costs in this sort of case-by-case decision making, as well as possible psychic costs. As Lazear has noted in a later article, "Few production environments lend themselves to costless and perfect measurement."[11] Moreover, there would be transaction costs for individual decision making. For example, if case-by-case decisions were permitted, there would be potential union objections based on fear of employer favoritism or arbitrariness.

The Puzzle of No Renegotiation

Why, in Lazear's model, do firms not individually renegotiate with employees who wish to continue work past the usual retirement age? A similar transaction-cost or information-cost argument, providing a partial explanation of the phenomenon, was suggested by Sidford Brown.[12] Assuming a continuous distribution of the reservation wage of such workers, then if one assumed a continuous wage function which employers would be willing to offer workers, that would imply no discrete change in the number of workers voluntarily retiring at any point in time or at any given age. But Lazear's theory provides a discontinuous wage function: the discontinuity occurs at time T, the usual retirement age. After time T the employer would be willing to pay a worker no more than his VMP, which by assumption is less than the wage paid at time T. A number of workers would choose voluntarily to retire at time T, specifically all those workers whose reservation wage was between $W(T)$ and $VMP(T)$. If it were true that the number who wished to retire for this reason was close to the total number of workers retirable under the mandatory retirement policy, the absence of renegotiation might then be reasonable. The costs incurred in offering renegotiation to all workers might not be justified if there were only a small number of workers with whom employment conditions could be successfully renegotiated.

The Veil of Ignorance

A routinization hypothesis offers another explanation of nonrenegotiation, a theory related to Lapp's insurance model.[13] Lapp sees employees as insuring themselves against random variations in productivity due to health loss or obsolescence of skills: they agree to an implicit contract with a pre-specified wage pattern consistent with the worker's expected VMP. Lapp assumes mandatory retirement is set at the age when most workers suffer a productivity decline.

Generalizing Lapp's model, however, there is no reason to assume that there is a prespecified wage pattern, merely that the worker might prefer to work in a firm where wages are set by job classification and seniority rather than one where his actual productivity will be monitored to set an individual wage. Workers might agree to an arrangement covering both those better and less well endowed, while still in ignorance as to the class in which they, when older, would belong. (The argument bears some family resemblance to Rawls' "veil of ignorance.")[14]

Lapp's theory (like Lazear's) argues that at mandatory retirement age, the firm forces the individual to leave employment rather than offer a reduced wage because of the likelihood of the offer being rejected.[15] This argument seems unpersuasive: it is not clear from the theory why there were not wage plans under which wages increased until (say) age 62 or 65, following which some older workers would want to stay with the firm but lose seniority protection against lay-off. Alternately, a "negative seniority" rule would provide that wages and relative job preference uniformly decline after that age. Such a plan would be prohibited now under the ADEA; perhaps unions previously resisted introducing the principle that wages could drop with time at the firm, or that seniority could decrease as well as rise.

Wage Rigidity

The nonrenegotiation of older workers' compensation can be analyzed as an instance of wage rigidity.[16] Three categories of explanation of the general phenomenon of wage rigidity have been identified by Flanagan.[17] Baily, for example, assumes employees are *risk averse* and therefore reach a deal with employers providing them wage insurance against changes in the economic "weather."[18] The argument might be generalized to the veil of ignorance argument, mentioned above, involving employees' risk aversion to possible unusual decline in their own abilities. In the *contracting* literature, difficulties in specifying and monitoring lead the parties to implicit understandings.[19] It is simple to extend this analysis to provide an explanation of retirement policies in terms of preference for a nonmonitored atmosphere. In the *principal-agent* literature, Lazear, for example, argues that the purpose of implicit contracts is to provide performance incentives to career employees.[20] Lazear has himself applied such an analysis to explain mandatory retirement.

Automatic Retirement

Some firms utilize age-work policies characterized by nonrenegotiation and nondiscretionary, tied-hands policies. These firms, in lieu of a so-called compulsory retirement policy that reserves employer discretion to retain a worker past the normal retirement age, adopt instead an automatic policy that permits no exceptions.[21] Even under compulsory retirement policies, it may be rare to renegotiate an adjustment of wages after the normal retirement age, but under automatic policies the practice is forbidden. Of active workers covered by mandatory retirement plans in 1974, 6.9 million were in plans calling only for compulsory retirement and 2 million were in plans providing only for automatic retirement. (Others were in plans providing some mix, or providing for forced early retirement.)[22] Thomas C. Shelling devoted his 1983 Richard T. Ely Lecture to considering the paradox of someone who attempts "to restrict her own options in violation of what she knows will be her preference at the time the behavior is to take place." Schelling noted, "It is not a phenomenon that fits easily into a discipline concerned with rational decision, revealed preference, and optimization over time."[23] He preferred to discuss the phenomenon as if an individual had several selves; certainly that explanation is more than a metaphor when analyzing organizational behavior.

When the automatic policy exists, even if the firm and employee both conclude that the productivity of an individual older worker and his own satisfaction justify his continued employment at the current wage, the tied-hands aspect of the policy forces the employer to retire the worker. If a mandatory policy is based on the use of age as a proxy for lower productivity, an employer with an automatic policy is applying an irrebuttable presumption of lack of capacity to an individual who in fact may be able to prove his continued worth. Such were the situations of police officer Murgia and foreign service officer Bradley, in the Supreme Court's mandatory retirement cases; both met the relevant standards of required productivity but were nevertheless retired because of age.[24] To the extent that this result is not explained by a theory of retirement (such as Lazear's analysis) its rationale is unsatisfactory.[25]

I have been arguing that there seems to be no rational reason for firms to enforce an automatic retirement rule that would deny themselves the option of retaining desirable older employees and renegotiating wages or other conditions of employment if necessary. Indeed, there is some research showing that firms do not always enforce such automatic self-denying rules, even if they are on the books. Rowe and Paine reported indications that supposedly mandatory rules for retirement were not enforced.[26]

Productivity Too Low or Wages Too High?

Lazear's theory implies that firms with mandatory retirement pay older workers more than do firms without mandatory retirement. Cohn, however, cites data showing that firms which have mandatory retirement do *not* in fact pay older workers higher wages than other firms.[27]

By assumption, however, firms with mandatory retirement must calculate the ratio of perceived productivity to wages for older workers as a lower one than nonretirement firms calculate. Cohn thus concludes that since these firms are not paying older workers higher wages, they must believe that older employees are less productive than younger employees. Indeed, Juanita Kreps's study showed that three-fourths of the mandatory retirement firms, but only one-eighth of the flexible retirement firms, believed that older workers are less productive.[28] And *The Older American Worker* study of employers' reasons for age-work policies (including reasons for limited hiring of older workers) gave productivity-related items 56.9 percent of the time, while compensation-related items were given only 16.6 percent of the time.[29] The first group included physical requirements, skills and experience, educational requirements, adaptability, training costs, quantity of work, speed in attaining proficiency, and personal characteristics; the second group included earnings, pension plan, and health and life insurance.

A 1982 study concluded that older workers' wage rates actually decline. The calculation, based on a longitudinal sample of men aged 45–64 running from 1966 to 1975, estimated that employee wage rates begin to decline in the sixth decade of life, at an amount under 1 percent per year during the fifties and at about 2 percent annually after the age of 60. This decline was masked by an overall increase in wage levels during this period, so the average real income did not drop.[30] These findings, like Cohn's, tend to contradict Lazear's age-bonus thesis, though they are incomplete because they do not separately analyze retirement and nonretirement firms.[31] Similarly, Boyle and associates, studying a sample of mature male wage earners, found that age has a significant negative impact on wages for jobs in the core sector of the economy, though it has no significant impact in the periphery. They concluded that ageism is more prevalent in core industries.[32]

These findings tend to undercut the age-bonus theory, and suggest that some other explanation of mandatory retirement is at work, perhaps a version of substantive or systemic rationality.

7 • The Union Choice Theory

A different explanation of mandatory retirement looks to union rather than employer choice. The influence of unions is often mentioned as a cause of age-work policies. In the weaker version of the hypothesis, the union acquiesces. If we assume that (for whatever reason) an employer strongly wished to have mandatory retirement and a union exists as bargaining agent, there is reason for the union to accept the employer proposal. It could then obtain quid pro quos, including a private pension plan to maintain the standard of living of its older members. The correlation of union membership, mandatory retirement, and pension coverage is thus understandable.[1] More difficult to explain, however, is the phenomenon of the unions' position: there are data indicating that even among employees *without* pension coverage, union employees are more than twice as likely to face mandatory retirement as are nonunion employees.[2] These data suggest a stronger version of the hypothesis: that unions actively seek the mandatory retirement system.

Alternative Explanations

One way of explaining this phenomenon would be to reason that unionization is correlated with larger size of firm and so is a proxy variable for firm type; association of large size and mandatory retirement would thus be explained. Another strategy would be to argue that unions bargain for seniority systems and that mandatory retirement is associated with such systems. If neither explanation suffices, some other account must be sought as to why unions sometimes accept mandatory retirement policies even without accompanying private pensions.

A third possible explanation is that a mandatory retirement policy advances the interests of the union officials rather than that of the current union membership. Cohn presents data to reject this alternative, accepting instead the explanation that union policy is consistent with its membership's attitude. His data so indicate in a weak fashion: more union employees than nonunion (49% compared to 36%) feel that "older workers should retire early to make room for others,"[3] though still fewer than a majority of union members so believe, and the question does not deal with *mandatory* retirement.

A fourth, and intuitively plausible, explanation for such union contracts would be intergroup competition between young and old union members. Many argue that the existence of such conflicts among workers may lead a union to wish to provide entry-level or promotional opportunities for younger workers and thus to support mandatory retirement. Younger union members will be constituents longer than older ones will, so perhaps union officials may choose to favor the interests of the younger ones, *ceteris paribus*.[4] It seems more plausible, however, that union officials will reflect the interests of whichever age group is currently a larger part of their membership. It is not entirely obvious, moreover, which union members favor mandatory retirement. Each member will have to balance increased promotional opportunities now against fewer years to enjoy those promotions at career's end. In general, younger workers will be more likely to strike this balance in favor of mandatory retirement than will older workers, as older workers have fewer promotional opportunities to look forward to. But it is not clear where the dividing line will fall, or on which side of that line a majority of union members will find themselves.

Personnel policies sought or accepted by unions may be motivated in part by relative concern for older and younger workers. The compulsory retirement policies of the Depression era are widely viewed as having been means of rationing scarce jobs in favor of younger workers.[5] Similarly, in the early 1960s, in the rapidly automating auto industry, union contracts provided substantially improved benefits for early retirees who withdrew from the work force. These provisions "reflected attitudes frequently voiced by auto workers in 1963 and 1964: early retirement was a high priority goal, and could be used as a means to reduce unemployment among younger workers."[6] Another example is the West Coast Longshoreman's Agreement of 1961, which accepted new work rules requiring fewer workers in exchange for early retirements, substantial dismissal pay for those short of retirement age, and enhanced unemployment benefits.[7] On the other hand, during the labor shortages of World War II and the 1950s, older workers were retained past "compulsory" retirement age.[8]

There are data indicating that older workers support mandatory retirement, which suggests that intergroup competition is not a sufficient explanation for the union's position. Dramatic data in one study show that, among union members, the percentage favoring retirement to make room for others is greater among older workers (over age 50) than among younger ones (52% versus 46%).[9] It may well be that union members have more fraternal feelings toward fellow workers than do nonunion members, but on the surface it is harder to understand why older union workers especially should be altruistic. One might suspect that the answers of older union members to the survey reflect a combination of fraternal feeling and some attribute linked with age. On one hypothesis, that attribute would be diminished job satisfaction, leading to a wish to retire for other than the stated reason, and linked with older age rather than with union membership. There is little evidential support, however, for such diminished job satisfaction as a basis for older workers' willingness to give up their jobs.

A more recent study of the general population is consistent with the hypothesis that some attribute linked with older age is also associated with willingness to give up jobs. Fifty percent of those age 65 and over agree (with 44% disagreeing) that older people should retire when they can "to give younger people more of a chance on the job," while among those 18 to 54 years old, only 31% agree (with 66% disagreeing).[10] These figures, however, may result from a cohort effect. Or older workers themselves may believe that age causes a typical decline in capacities and so may accept retirement more easily.[11] The figures for *non*union members in the study used by Cohn do not show an increase in support for retirement among older as compared to younger workers, failing to support this hypothesis.[12]

An alternative explanation for the position of older union members is that the group of older workers (over age 50) includes two subgroups: those close to retirement age (say, age 60–65), and those close to age 50 (say, age 50–59). Maybe the relatively younger group of workers are the ones who benefit from increased promotional opportunity; they are next in line for the jobs now held by the 65-year-olds.

Cohn's further explanation of the union phenomenon is that unions wish to increase the total number of union members (actives plus veterans) in order to maximize their political power.[13] The increase in power of the union gained through such a policy is apparently thought to inure to the benefit of all its members, so that each individual by accepting his own mandatory retirement hopes to maximize the lifetime total of his wages and the members' shared political influence. This explanation would represent another instance of intertemporal choice, an individual's allocation of work, leisure, and other values over a life cycle. Intuitively, the explanation seems quite doubtful.

Another way of dealing with the supposed union phenomenon would be to conclude that it is a pseudophenomenon, except in special circumstances when younger workers have had to compete against older ones for particularly scarce jobs. Unions have not in fact generally sought mandatory retirement policies. There is a variety of data showing union facilitation of continued work by older workers, either at standard rates or at lower wages matching their presumed diminished productivity. According to an early-twentieth-century report of the U.S. Commissioner of Labor, many local unions at that time had maintained for many years policies permitting older members to work for a wage rate lower than the rate fixed for younger members. In some local unions the member had been permitted to fix his own wage rate, the only condition being that he observe union rules.[14] Older workers dismissed from their jobs in that era generally remained in the work force, though frequently encountering difficulty in obtaining new positions and sometimes having to switch from higher-paying jobs to work as unskilled laborers.[15]

Similarly, a survey of international unions at mid-century reported by Abrams showed that 60 percent permitted older workers to take lower-rated jobs at lower wage rates; 30 percent refused to do so; 10 percent left it to locals.[16] At that time, almost all the internationals prohibited older workers from staying in their regular jobs at a lower rate matching decreased productivity, and even downgrading was often opposed in practice by unions.

Pension policies, along with other fringe benefits, were encouraged under the World War II wage stabilization programs and stimulated by a 1948 decision of the National Labor Relations Board holding that they were compulsory subjects of bargaining for employers.[17] During the 1940s and early 1950s, unions often bargained to push up mandatory retirement ages or to abolish them entirely if possible.[18] In some firms, unions were successful in securing a flexible retirement policy for their members, even though nonunion workers in the same firms were subject to an involuntary plan. Company policy sometimes prevailed over union opposition, while involuntary retirement was only sometimes accepted by the union.[19] In collectively bargained pension plans in the early 1950s, unions were virtually unanimous in opposition to compulsory retirement; the greater the degree of union participation in administering the plans, the less likely a mandatory feature.[20] The 1963 and 1965 AFL-CIO Constitutional Conventions called for investigation of rigid systems of forced retirement of older workers and for legislation curtailing discrimination based on age. The AFL pension handbook opposed compulsory retirement.[21] Further, mandatory retirement provisions are less common in plans negotiated by unions (less than 40%) than in other plans (more than 70%).[22] These data suggest that the supposed phenomenon of the unions' position may be contrafactual, and thus requires no explanation.

Collective Decision Making: Nonmonitored Atmosphere

In a theory similar to that of union choice, Gunderson and Pesando conclude that the mandatory retirement system arises from labor-management trade-offs and can be both an efficient and an equitable work rule, achieved via collective decision making.[23] They quickly reject as unfounded the argument that mandatory retirement opens up new jobs for the young. They also doubt two assumptions inherent in legislation against mandatory retirement: that mandatory retirement often is an externally imposed constraint not reflecting in any fashion the preferences of individual workers, and that what emerges from labor-management trade-offs is somehow socially undesirable. "The reasons for this presumed market failure . . . are seldom made explicit in the current debate." Their contention is that the various mandatory retirement policies are better regarded as "endogenous institutional responses to labour-management trade offs, constrained by legitimate market pressures" as well as by societal pressures expressed through legislation and public policy.[24]

Gunderson and Pesando argue that "the fact that mandatory retirement has emerged in response to market forces merits emphasis." The root of their argument is "the fact" that the mandatory retirement age "has emerged in response to the interplay of market forces," which "suggests that it has a rationale in terms of the efficient utilization of human resources."[25] They add: "In essence the argument . . . rests on the belief that the individual parties themselves are best able to determine this one element in the total package of compensation and work rules. Their collective decision can be regarded as an endogenous institutional response to their own various trade offs and to the legitimate concerns of the other parties."[26] Their economic case for mandatory retirement rests on the possibility that both firms and workers can in principle be made better off by entering into implicit or explicit contracts that may, at times, limit their freedom.

What workers seek in such bargaining, according to Gunderson and Pesando, is what we call a nonmonitored atmosphere. A mandatory retirement system has a psychological payoff for older workers. It shields them from employer monitoring and termination systems, loss of anonymity, wage adjustments, and peer-group pressure to maintain productivity. Gunderson and Pesando thus emphasize that psychological attitudes in labor-management relations have a causal role in the adoption of mandatory retirement.

In a footnote, these authors state that the extent to which the concerns of the various parties, especially minority groups, are given "adequate" weight in the give-and-take of the negotiation process is a subject in need of further research.[27] They thus implicitly leave as an open question whether the aged minority is "adequately" represented. They think it a sensible policy to allow everyone to retire early and to hire back the most productive on a contractual basis. But they do not explain why many firms deny themselves such a "sensible" arrangement; thus, their study is incomplete.

8 • Statistical Discrimination Theories

The substantive rationality explanation of mandatory retirement is logically premised on the conclusion of some employers that the perceived marginal productivity of older workers does not justify their marginal wages. This belief alone would not lead logically to adoption of a mandatory retirement policy; it must be supplemented by the process rationality judgment that age-based generalization is a more efficient method of personnel decision than individualized determination. One version of a process rationality scenario is discussed in this chapter: the adoption of mandatory retirement because of the belief that older workers are generally less productive can be explained in terms of *statistical discrimination*. The profit-maximizing employer will discriminate against blacks or women or older workers if they are regarded as less productive *on the average* than younger white men, *and* if the cost of gaining information on individual applicants is high. Thurow uses this terminology; Phelps introduced the statistical theory of discrimination to account for racial and sexual discrimination in the labor market; and Arrow independently invented the theory.[1]

Definitions

Theories of statistical discrimination use the word *discriminate* nonpejoratively, in its root meaning of "distinguish." Ramm defines the difference between discrimination in its pejorative and neutral senses in that the former involves an "unfair" difference. He gives age discrimination as an example: so long as distinctions because of age are generally accepted, we regard them as neutral. If, however, the attitude toward old age changes and if, for example, old employees are dismissed more often than young workers, then there is discrimination in the pejorative sense of the word.[2] Becker, taking a different viewpoint, defines discrimination as "an employer's treatment of an employee that is based on considerations *other than productivity*."[3]

One may usefully distinguish between group discrimination and individual discrimination.[4] They are both subcategories of *economic discrimination,* defined as existing when equal productivity is not rewarded with equal pay (similar to Becker's usage). *Group discrimination* exists when the average wage of a group is not proportional to its average productivity. *Individual discrimination* exists when individual workers, within a group, are not paid according to their true ability. Applied to the situation of mandatory retirement, group discrimination can be said to exist if the employer is using a mistaken generalization; older workers then would be forced to retire at an age when, on the average, they still are productive enough to justify their wages. Even if the generalization were correct, however, there would be some individual older workers who are still highly productive while an average worker of the same age is not. To apply the accurate generalization to that individual would be individual discrimination. The statistical discrimination theory argues that, where group differences in productivity exist in fact, individual discrimination will occur if there are not adequate and inexpensive methods to measure true individual productivity.

Posner and Thurow

The statistical discrimination hypothesis is discussed by Richard Posner, whose use of the theory has special legal salience because of his influence as a scholar of Law and Economics and as a judge of the U.S. Court of Appeals.[5] Posner has discussed statistical discrimination in legal contexts, where proxy characteristics that in themselves are irrelevant (racial and ethnic identity) are correlated with characteristics that are considered relevant. He regards such action as identical to *prejudice,* which he defines as the ascription of relevant attributes to all members of a group, where the group is defined in terms of some proxy characteristic. The relevant attributes are in fact frequently but not always possessed by members of that group; the ascription is made without individualized determination, and sometimes without even willingness to consider evidence that the individual does not have the relevant characteristic.

Posner argues that to the extent an attribute difficult to conceal (like race or ethnic identity) is correlated with desired or undesired characteristics, it is rational to use the first attribute as a proxy for the underlying characteristic with which it is correlated. The costs due to error in using the proxy may be smaller than the information costs of making a more extensive sampling. Discrimination may thus be economically efficient. Posner regards it to be relatively rare that prejudice is based on characteristics in fact not common in a group; in that sense, he regards most prejudice as "rational."[6] He emphasizes, however, that the practice when applied to racial groups may contravene distributive social policies and thus be condemnable.

Thurow defines statistical discrimination as occurring whenever individuals are judged on the basis of the average characteristics of the group or groups to which they belong rather than upon their personal characteristics. Justified statistical discrimination in Thurow's sense thus produces unjustified individual discrimination. Certain disfavored groups of employees are evaluated by employers in a statistically discriminatory manner. "The judgments are correct, factual, and objective in the sense that the group actually has the characteristics that are ascribed to it, but the judgments are incorrect with respect to many individuals within the group."[7] If statistical discrimination did explain mandatory retirement, by Thurow's definition it would be because employers are correct in estimating the usual age-related decline in productivity. But since the data summarized in Part 3 of this work suggest many employers are in error when making those estimates, then we should say it is (unjustified) group discrimination rather than merely individual discrimination that is at work.

Job Competition

Thurow's analysis makes a distinction between wage and job competition.[8] Assuming on the one hand that wage competition exists, a job applicant who belongs to a disfavored group will be hired at a lower wage because of his supposed production characteristics. Once the worker is on the job, however, he can demonstrate that he has the right production characteristics regardless of the group to which he belongs, and his wage will then rise to the level of others with the right characteristics. Assuming on the other hand that job competition exists, the individual who belongs to a group with a higher probability of having the undesired production characteristic is not hired, and thus has no way to demonstrate that he himself has the desired characteristics. Thurow believes that job competition, rather than wage competition, is prevalent: employers make an all-or-nothing decision whether to hire. His model supplies a concept to describe the nonhiring phenomenon and the absence of renegotiation: both can be characterized as a matter of job rather than wage competition. By the job competition assumption, the employer who believes that the elderly are usually not as able as the young will not adjust wages or conditions of employment in order to hire and retain older workers, because she makes all-or-nothing hiring decisions.

Thurow's version of statistical discrimination does not, however, explain the generalization phenomenon as to retirement of older workers. Nor does the theory successfully explain the absence of renegotiation, though supplying a label for it. By hypothesis the older worker is already on the job and has exhibited his own personal characteristics. A firm deciding about retaining older workers can actually observe their revealed individual productivity. Why would that firm prefer to evaluate older workers in terms of the presumed characteristics of their age group? The Thurow analysis by itself supplies no general explanation.

Process Rationality

Process rationality hypotheses explain the generalization phenomenon with the assumption that productivity is hard to measure. According to the Phelps-Arrow version of the theory the explanation is more adequate if the identification of individual workers' productivities is difficult while age-related decline can be observed in general. Individual case-by-case evaluation is costly: there are information costs, transaction costs, psychic costs, and union objections.

Even so, some other proxy characteristics, such as overall health, might be better predictors.[9] Though health would be more difficult than age to establish in a noncontestable way, tests for overall health are nonetheless available. And it also remains necessary to explicate the ratchet effect to show why, even if employers have a rational reason to treat all workers at a given age alike, they make job rather than wage decisions and use mandatory retirement rather than a declining wage schedule.

The statistical discrimination theory as applied to the elderly assumes that employees' productivity characteristics do typically begin to decline in their mid-sixties but that the change is hard to measure in individual cases.

The assumed difficulties in measurement and decline in productivity need not be general ones. Individual productivity can be difficult to measure in situations requiring cooperative effort by a group of people. Perhaps decline past acceptable limits commonly occurs in workers in some industries and for some positions. Those employers might correctly believe it would be too difficult for them to make accurate, fair, and justifiable individualized determinations of appropriate retirement age; they could reasonably be expected to use age-based generalizations. In some situations such employers might even justify age-work policies as a bona fide occupational qualification under the Age Discrimination in Employment Act.[10]

Another hypothesis is that in some industries and for some positions, the employee's own decision to retire voluntarily may be less closely correlated with decline in productivity than in other industries and positions. Perhaps some types of firms need to use mandatory retirement because workers there do not voluntarily retire when their productivity fails. Employees' retirement decisions are heavily influenced by reasons other than their productivity (particularly health and pension benefits).[11]

In one survey of employers, the reason most frequently given for involuntary retirement policies was that a uniform policy avoids the disadvantages of distinguishing between employees, a process rationality explanation. Individual decisions were regarded as both hard to make and hard to explain.[12] A related hypothesis is that in situations where productivity can be observed to decline *before* the mandatory retirement age in the individual case, firms with a "usual" retirement age are willing to make temporary accommodations and retain workers until that age.[13]

In summary, if one accepts statistical discrimination as an explanation, one must still propound a detailed mechanism explaining the phenomena of absence of renegotiation and generalization. It must be shown for particular jobs and industries why wages are not adjusted individually and why individual retention decisions are not made instead of retiring all older workers. Thurow's hypothesis of job competition describes nonnegotiation; it does not, however, suffice to explain the generalization phenomenon as to mandatory retirement.

The Ratchet Effect

Workers are unlikely to accept easily an employer's decision to reduce wages; there is a ratchet effect, a stickiness in downward wage adjustments.[14] Boskin has argued that the difficulties of reducing wages "when productivity drops late in life—due to physical problems or obsolescence of technological knowledge and skills" may be "a major reason" why mandatory retirement policies were adopted in the first place.[15]

It is not self-evident, though, that workers would more readily accept an employer's discharge decision than a wage cut; data on this point was presented above (Chapter 6). Cohn comments that where private pensions exist, they soften the blow of retirement; presumably he believes that workers would prefer to do no work and receive a pension than to continue to work at reduced wages. His assumption is one of an intertemporal choice of a certain mix of work, wages, and leisure. But this explanation still does not connect the employee's intertemporal choice with the employer's decision to institute mandatory retirement.

There is a related economic explanation based on the opportunity costs of working. If hefty pensions offering a high replacement ratio are available, the vast majority of covered workers might prefer to fall back on their pensions than to continue to work at a cut in pay. If only a few employees would prefer to accept the pay cut and continue working, then, especially in large firms or unionized industries, it might not be worth the time and costs of working out and bickering over the appropriate declining wage schedule. This is the Sidford Brown explanation given above.

The statistical discrimination studies expound possible models stating that, in theory, it is possible that age-based personnel decisions might be economically efficient. These models generally do not have sufficient supporting empirical data for particular jobs or firms.

Categorical Discrimination

Crocker and Snow have analyzed a related issue, considering *categorical discrimination* in the insurance industry. There, some observable trait is used to categorize individuals.[16] By hypothesis, the observable trait is not of itself relevant, but the trait that is important is unobservable, and the observable trait is "correlated with, and hence informative about" the unobservable one. They differentiate between categorization which is costless, that which is somewhat costly, and that which is quite costly. Hoy has shown that the market generally uses costless categorization but that whether doing so maximizes overall benefits is uncertain, since there are losers as well as winners from such a system.[17] Crocker and Snow demonstrate the possibility of a system under which costless categorization can be employed so that no one loses. When categorization is costly, however, the market may categorize even when the savings to winners is less than the costs to losers. They conclude:

> [I]f the cost of categorization is large enough the market does not categorize, which is efficient. If the cost is small enough the market does categorize, which is again efficient since the winners from categorization could compensate the losers. However, for intermediate levels of cost the market still categorizes even though the winners from categorization could not compensate the losers. We conclude that the market can be an inefficient mechanism for allocating resources to the acquisition of information.[18]

This analysis provides an interesting analogy to the question of using age as a proxy for productivity in categorizing employees. One is tempted to think that age is a costless categorization (Crocker and Snow regard it as such), usable as an imperfect proxy for productivity, and thus that Crocker and Snow's conclusions apply to the economic efficiency of categorizing employees by age for personnel decisions. Under their reasoning, the market may produce age-based decision making even when it is economically inefficient to do so. Moreover, the imperfectness of age as a proxy means that in individual instances, the age-based decision will harm productivity by excluding productive workers. Age-based personnel decisions may also entail deadweight losses owing to bad effects on morale. Use of age to measure productivity, as opposed to its use in the insurance market, is thus not cost-free. Furthermore, while the insurance analysis assumes that the trait of real interest (e.g., the actual likelihood that the individual will die that year) is unobservable, in the employment situation the key trait (say, productivity) is generally observable. In the employment situation, use of categorical discriminations by age must be compared to other forms of decision making. There are always other proxies available to measure productivity (say, physical exams). Even the conclusion that in theory categorical discrimination by age might be efficient does not show that in the real world it is more efficient than readily available alternatives.

9 • Sociological Theories

We turn now from the work of economists to that of sociologists and historians. Not all these studies directly address the causal questions of central concern to this study. While some have discussed causes of mandatory retirement, others deal with retirement in general, aging, or the place of the elderly in society. These studies nevertheless point to a rejection of simple versions of economic rationality as a sufficient causal explanation for mandatory retirement.

Cultural History

To understand mandatory retirement in America, it is helpful to place it in the context of the larger history of the cultural conception of the elderly and their changing social role.

The role of the elderly has undergone a dramatic transformation during the course of American history, most scholars agree. But historians differ as to the extent of the changes, when they occurred, and to what extent the transformation was caused by changes in the economy, in the general society, and in cultural ideals. In *Growing Old In America,* Fischer argued that a major change in the relations between generations occurred between 1770 and 1820, and that it was part of a worldwide revolution in social values.[1] In colonial times old age was comparatively rare and, perhaps for that reason, it was highly respected. Seventeenth- and eighteenth-century literature taught people that they were expected to show the elderly deference and respect, even "veneration." The relationship was not only expected but thought to be biologically given. "The light of nature teacheth men to honour age. . . . In most civilized nations they have done so."[2] Behavior mirrored those attitudes, Fischer concluded. For example, in the most important public gatherings in New England—congregational worship—seats were assigned according to dignity, and the most honorable places went to the oldest rather than the richest or strongest.

Late in the eighteenth century, however, the most profound social revolution in modern history occurred, encompassing the American and French Revolutions and every area of human relations. This was the end of the *ancien régime,* and Fischer argues that it was also an end to the *régime des anciens.*

Age veneration was replaced by age equality or preference for youth. And so, instead of wigs and white powder to make men look old, there were hair dyes and tints to make them look young. Fischer also dates a new language to express contempt for old people to this period. In the middle of the nineteenth century words for the old which previously had had an honorific meaning acquired new pejorative usages; he cites the *Oxford English Dictionary* for changes during this period in the meaning of *gaffer, fogy, greybeard, old guard,* and *superannuated.* And he dates the first mandatory retirement rules to 1777–1818. Fischer's book cites much other evidence to support his conclusion that a revolution in attitudes toward the age occurred between 1770 and 1820. From 1820 to the present, the lines of change have been straight and stable, and the old have become displaced and despised.

Achenbaum, in *Old Age in the New Land,* agreed that early America respected the old for their experience, wisdom, and longevity, and that attitudes toward them changed in modern times from positive to negative.[3] He differed from Fischer in dating the change to 1865–1914 rather than to 1770–1820, making it post–Civil War rather than post-Revolution.

Other historians have argued, to the contrary, that in colonial America respect was based more on wealth than on longevity.[4] Some have also questioned whether there existed a later trend toward disrespect for the elderly. As an example of the diverse evidence they cite, a quantitative study of magazine articles from 1845 to 1882 found old persons still depicted as useful members of society, though less visible than the young.[5]

Notwithstanding these challenges to the historical change thesis, a large body of scholarship agrees that the typical life course of the elderly was different a century and more ago. The transition of an individual to a postadult status then occurred later than today, and at a less clear-cut point. For most people who lived that long, at different times after 65 there would be crucial turning points, such as the departure of the last child from home, the relinquishment of the status of head of household, and retirement.[6]

Carole Haber concludes that by the late nineteenth century a conception of the elderly as disabled and needy was widespread in the culture, though it was not accurate for most.[7] That view of the elderly as disabled was also propagated by the new profession of efficiency engineers. The adoption of mandatory retirement plans in the late nineteenth century reflected the understanding of the elderly as disabled. Serving to legitimate the removal of the elderly from the work force, mandatory retirement on a pension also helped employers cope with seniority and maintain employee discipline and was thought to provide jobs for the young.

The rise of mandatory retirement was thus consistent with overall trends in the vision held of the elderly in America, though details of the relationship may be hard to pinpoint, since scholars differ as to the causes, timing, and extent of those trends.

Modernization Theory

A number of works stress that economic and social changes have affected the elderly in diverse ways.[8] Some scholars have emphasized the effects of modernization (including the major economic changes of industrialization) on changes in the role of the elderly, and some analysts of these processes have used the sociological perspective of structural functionalism.[9] Burgess emphasized industrialization's effect in changing the position of the elderly.[10] He argued, for example, that mass production had decreased the number of self-employed entrepreneurs; the loss of decision-making power in the work place created pressures for retirement. Burgess's argument was developed by Cowgill, who analyzed along several lines of causation the effect that modernization—not just industrialization—had on the aged.[11] One factor was modern health technology, which prolonged the lives of workers. The death of older workers was thus postponed, and job openings were not created rapidly enough to accommodate the expanding pool of workers. The system of retirement was thus developed as a social substitute for death. Cowgill's conclusion was that longer life spans and declining birth rates, changing the distribution of the population by age, yielded increased intergenerational conflict for jobs.[12] His conclusion seems open to challenge.

A second line of causation, Cowgill argued, was that older workers would naturally be more heavily represented in the established occupations. Modern economic technology created new occupations and transformed most of the old ones, causing loss of jobs held by the aged. Furthermore, with the growth of mass education there was a lessened base for respect of the superior knowledge of the elderly. Younger workers were assumed by employers to be more suitable for the new jobs. There were reasons, then, for firms involuntarily to retire older workers.

Thus in modernization theory increased longevity heightened competitive pressures to force the aged out of desired positions, industrialization eliminated many jobs held by the aged, and mass education lessened the value of their experience. But Cowgill's theory did not seek to explain many characteristics of mandatory retirement.

"There is now an immense body of literature," Quadagno has pointed out, "that exists for the sole purpose of debunking modernization theory."[13] In modernization theory, demographic and technological changes are viewed as the causal factors, and the diminished modern social status of the aged is a result. The work of several social historians indicates that the arrow of causation flowed in the other direction. Well before population aging and industrialization occurred, there was a decline in the status of the elderly, which these social historians explain as part of a change in world view or ideology, from hierarchical traditional social organization to an egalitarian achievement-oriented one. The work of Fischer, Achenbaum, Haber, and Graebner all support this interpretation.[14]

There are other criticisms of modernization theory as an explanation for mandatory retirement. Haber claims that the aged were capable of filling the new urban jobs; women and children were hired for many of those new jobs. That the aged increasingly became unemployed thus requires further explanation beyond what modernization theory offers. Graebner points out that mandatory retirement did not begin in declining industries, those presumably overstocked with older workers. Fischer provides documentation to prove that in the industries that adopted mandatory retirement early, mechanization had not yet reduced the need for workers. Where there was a substantial oversupply of labor, direct intergenerational competition for jobs did not seem to play a major role in the adoption of mandatory retirement policies. Atchley's recent review concluded, "Thus none of the elements of modernization theory fits the facts about the development of retirement."[15]

Other Sociological Theories

Age Stratification

Riley, Johnson, and Foner developed a sociological viewpoint which uses as its explanatory concept the allocation by a culture of specific social roles to particular age stages.[16] Within each individual's life course, he or she moves from one stage to the next; each age cohort in turn takes on a succession of allocated roles. For example, we allocate education to the young and life's work to the next age stage. Age-stratification theory highlights the influence on retirement of informal pressures and normative ideas.

The theory does not attempt to explain most of the characteristics of mandatory retirement that have been identified in this study. Atchley offers the further criticism that retirement did not come to be viewed as "normative"—that is, as "a legitimate part of the life course rather than an unfortunate fact of some working lives"—until the 1960s, when financial security for the retiree became possible.[17] (Others have dated the change to the adoption of the Social Security System in the 1930s.) The rise of mandatory retirement practices before those developments thus remain unexplained.

Disengagement

Another sociological theory offering an explanation of retirement is Cumming's disengagement theory. Cumming's theory moves from a description of the gradual disengagement of the elderly from their social roles to a normative conclusion that such disengagement is functionally necessary. "When a middle-aged, fully-engaged person dies, he leaves many broken ties and disrupted situations. Disengagement [of the old from important social roles] thus frees the old to die without disrupting vital affairs." [18] Mandatory retirement is explained teleologically by its social function. Crucial social roles must be occupied by the middle-aged, not the elderly. Were these roles to be filled by a group with a high death rate, too much disruption would occur when fully engaged people die.

Cumming's theory would lead to the conclusion that aged leaders, more than holders of ordinary jobs, should be required to retire. And indeed many earlier age-work policies did apply only to executives. [19] But there are also facts to the contrary. Mandatory retirement began, for example, with ordinary railroad workers, and many crucial social positions were exempt from mandatory retirement. Similarly, disengagement theory would predict that at periods with a higher death rate of older persons, it would be more necessary to exclude the elderly from leadership positions. Again, the facts are to the contrary. During the colonial period in America, for example, though the death rates of the elderly were higher than they now are, leadership was more concentrated in older men than now. [20] The death rate for those in their sixties was lower while mandatory retirement flourished than it was in earlier generations when there was no such practice. Cumming's disengagement theory, not just its application to retirement, is now widely discredited.

Exchange

Dowd developed an exchange theory stating that those with fewer resources at their command will gain less in their social exchanges with others. [21] He argues that the aged are believed to have less to give, and so are given less. To Dowd, the use of age as a criterion—for mandatory retirement, among other practices—is age discrimination. Dowd does not explain the characteristics of mandatory retirement we have identified, nor does he indicate why many elderly workers were able to avoid mandatory retirement, nor does he discuss why many received valuable government and private pension benefits. Thus, the theory is insufficient.

Retirement as a Social Institution

A recent major sociological attempt to explain retirement deals with retirement as a social institution.[22] Robert Atchley's conclusion is that mandatory retirement arose initially as a solution to the problem of setting a limit on seniority rights to one's job and, as such, was produced through negotiations between unions and management. He traces the employer position seeking such limits to management's perception that the aged were less effective workers.[23] Atchley notes the existence of massive oversupplies of inexpensive labor as the context within which the firms' erroneous actions were taken. Presumably implicit in his theory is the argument that the oversupply insulated firms from market correction for their discharge of effective workers. He rejects intergenerational conflict *per se* as a causal factor, concluding that it had no major role in the evolution of retirement.

In Atchley's reading of history, mandatory retirement arose as management's answer to unions' insistence on seniority systems. Senior workers were more expensive than younger ones, and some of the senior workers would be "superannuated"—rendered ineffective because of the effects of aging. Mandatory retirement solved both problems. Atchley mentions in passing that employers sought relief from having to make judgments about superannuation. He also states that unions, while striving for seniority systems, were willing to trade off mandatory retirement because few workers then reached mandatory retirement age.[24] This last point seems weak: unions and management faced the same work force, and if there were enough older workers for the managers to care about and want to retire, there were enough for unions to care about and want to protect.

Atchley also argues that in earlier periods management simply rejected older workers on the erroneous belief they were less efficient. In more recent years the rationale for retirement shifted to the "control of unemployment and creation of job opportunities . . . the need to circulate a large labor force through a somewhat smaller array of jobs."[25] He does not develop the point or explicate the institutions through which the perceived need is mediated to affect decisions of individual employers. Presumably, it is through the negotiation postures of unions.

This theory places relatively less emphasis than some others on economic and demographic causal factors. Instead, special emphasis is given to social ideology—beliefs that devalued the contribution of older workers, serving as a basis for age discrimination in employment and including a pro-retirement attitude. Atchley also argues that new technologies reduced the need for labor and that labor surpluses and periodic high unemployment produced the motivation to find ways to reduce the size of the labor force. The previous capacity of work organizations to deal with disabled workers by reassignment to easier work was reduced by two factors: the increased numbers of workers living to old age and the standardization of jobs in large organizations.

Following Atchley, Malcolm Morrison develops a perception of retirement as a social institution. Writing in a 1986 volume, *Our Aging Society,* he sees the institution reflecting social organizations, ideologies and values, the alternatives established by the culture, and the rewards or constraints that influence choice among those alternatives. Morrison observes that "today's values and policies . . . generally exclude older people from social, economic and cultural participation in society." [26]

Like many of the arguments I have reviewed, Morrison's understanding of the causal chain is hard to determine. In Chapter 11 I will discuss extensive Labor Department studies on mandatory retirement on which Morrison worked. In his 1986 essay, what he seems to count as the root causes of change are a wide range of demographic, economic, political, and sociocultural circumstances, with industrialization as an underlying cause. In his conception, the range of causes produce social values, expectations, and beliefs. A major reason for the current lowered participation of the elderly in the work force is a set of beliefs, now entrenched, that assume decline, redundancy, and dependency on their part—beliefs not reflecting their actual capacities.

Morrison identifies several aspects of industrial development, beginning during the latter half of the nineteenth century, as precursors of retirement. First, a social insurance ideology developed to support a role for government in providing income security for wage earners. Bismarck articulated the new ideology which led to national old-age pension systems that made possible and legitimated retirement.

Moreover, pension plans were initiated by the military and judicial sectors of the U.S. government and by a small number of private companies; most of the plans required compulsory retirement. Pensions, however, were still considered unusual in the early period. (Morrison reasons that it is the increasing availability of public and private resources that has led to an early retirement trend in the United States and many other developed nations.)

Economic problems, such as widespread unemployment caused by cyclical business conditions, effected further economic deprivation in old age. Industrial unions emerged and tried to establish job security systems based on seniority, protecting many older workers from layoff. Management accepted seniority systems in return for the unions' acceptance of uniform mandatory retirement rules "for workers considered to have reached an age of diminished productivity." That trade "was originally perceived primarily as a protection for senior (and older) workers."[27]

"General expectations that employees would continue working until stopped by ill health, debilitation, or death" continued for some time, largely unaffected by the ideology of state responsibility for income security for the aged, the few private pension plans, or the seniority system.[28] But stereotypes about older workers' productivity became major factors. Between 1920 and 1940, during a period of rapid industrialization and labor-intensive employment expansion, negative stereotypes developed about older employees, related to a "wear-and-tear" theory of older workers. "Scientific management techniques" concentrating on speed of work were adopted in the new industrial bureaucracies. The assumption was that a worker's lifetime productive capacity was relatively fixed and that it would be exhausted over time. While intense speed would get the most out of an employee's capacity, it would also increase stress, which it was assumed would result in an absolute decline in productive capacity with age. "Although there was never much objective support for beliefs about the relationship between age and declining capacities," these negative stereotypes have persisted and have hardened with additional unfavorable assumptions about skill obsolescence, reduced learning capacity, resistance to change, and slower decision making with aging.[29] Older employees, presumably worn out, could easily be replaced with an increasing immigrant labor supply or through automation.

Morrison cites John Myles for the theory that the institution of retirement is to be understood in the context of industrial capitalism. The new managerial class supported the development of retirement policies permitting greater control over the composition and movement of the labor force.[30] This theory, Morrison explains, "suggests that the retirement institution was primarily a response to the requirements of industrial capitalism, which demanded policies of 'superannuation' based on the view that older workers were unable to maintain their productivity, and thus created production inefficiency."[31]

While recognizing the positive values of retirement, Morrison questions whether it is a good social policy to limit the overall productivity of as much as 20 percent of the population. He recommends the goal of achieving enough flexibility for older persons to remain productive, whether this flexibility comes about through a redefinition of retirement or through the recognition of a "new life-cycle period as a flexible and multi-option stage for older persons."[32]

Industrialization in England

Most of the studies reviewed here concern the United States. There is, however, a recent study of the growth of retirement in nineteenth-century England, part of Quadagno's book, *Aging in Early Industrial Society.* In England, as in the United States, "retirement as a general concept did not appear until the closing years of the nineteenth century."[33] The 1891 census was the first that listed the retired as a separate category (though the concept then included younger workers who were physically or mentally incapacitated).[34]

Though Quadagno is more interested in the beginning of pensions, her work contains some clues relating to the rise of mandatory retirement. In early industrial England, age-work practices were common. "There can be no doubt as to the difficulty experienced on the part of men engaged in certain occupations to obtain employment as their age increases," concluded a contemporaneous report on unemployment.[35]

Though Quadagno does not organize her discussion in this way, we can distill from it five reasons for the development of mandatory retirement in England at the end of the nineteenth century. All her reasons involve what I call substantive rationality. She devotes a major section to considering the hypothesis that industrialization was the key factor in phasing older workers out of the labor force and ends up questioning any simple explanation based on technological changes. Older workers were disproportionately represented in declining occupations, but she finds that the main effect of that fact was that they entered the new occupations less than younger men did. The new technology did have a negative effect on the aged in those traditional occupations that became mechanized, such as weaving: "In this case, older workers who were employed as wage laborers were unable to acquire new skills that would allow them to compete successfully against younger workers."[36] She does not explain why the old dogs could not learn new tricks.

Quadagno also mentions an economically rational reaction by employers to the Workman's Compensation Act. Although this act was a reform measure intended to compensate industrial workers for injuries on the job, it led many employers to force older workers out because the elderly were believed more likely to be injured on the job.[37] Quadagno does not refer to the studies of actual injury rates but accepts the employers' belief as accurate.

Her third explanation is based on a diminished productivity-wage ratio under various industrial conditions: "As firms grew larger and the workplace became the factory, it was increasingly less efficient to keep older workers around for the few odd chores they might perform."[38] She gives no basis for her conclusions about efficiency or productivity, but presumedly reflects the views employers held. She does note that continued employment of the elderly was sometimes functional for the firm. Practice varied from one manufacturer to another. Reduced pay for reduced work occurred through piecework. As a contemporary put it, "In piecework trades so long as men can maintain the standards of quality of the article they produce, the employers are prepared to allow them to go on, knowing that any loss of speed falls upon the men and not the employers."[39] Moreover, in some industries, the aged did remain employed working at reduced hourly wage rates for odd jobs.

In many firms, however, unions, fearful of jeopardizing their newly gained wage guarantees, objected to the practice of employing older workers at lower wage rates. For example, one trade unionist testified before a Royal Commission: "[W]e have to remember this, that if we allowed that man, when he arrived at a certain age to work for less wages than what may be termed the strong and lusty, the employers would at once take the opportunity of causing a downward tendency to the wages of the general body of workmen."[40] The logic underlying this reasoning is not developed. If the elderly were as productive as the young, it is unclear why they would not be paid full rate. If, as assumed by both the unions and Quadagno, the elderly were less productive, then paying them a lower rate should not have affected the rate of the more able. Whatever the logical force of the reasoning, the combination of the employers' judgment that the elderly were less productive, and union resistance to lower rates, reduced the work opportunities for older workers.

The final explanation Quadagno offers is also based on economic changes, though mediated through changed conceptions. Associated with the developments in the form of industrial organization, there was an alteration in the cultural climate as to the responsibilities of business to its older workers. Traditional businesses had been more paternalistic and felt a responsibility to elderly workmen; new managers did not. One representative of a Friendly Society testified: "So far as private firms are concerned, there is very great sympathy with the old workmen, and I believe that masters in the district I came from do their best to find such employment [for the elderly]. But so far as [incorporated] firms are concerned . . . well, the same sympathy is not experienced and the same help is not afforded. One can well understand that, because the managers feel the responsibility to the shareholders and also the directors feel such responsibility."[41]

All Quadagno's explanations are based on what I call substantive rationality, and all assume that older workers were generally no longer sufficiently productive to continue working. If indeed this was not as uniformly true as employers then believed (and I set out in Part 3 the evidence that it was not), there is little in her discussion to explain the strength of the mistaken belief. Quadagno does not focus on involuntary retirement and does not consider the practice of retirement at a fixed age. Nevertheless, her study of the English historical evidence is of great interest for comparison with the United States, as it reveals the power of the conventional wisdom on older workers from a different data base.

10 • Histories of Retirement

Two narrative histories of the rise of retirement in America deserve special notice: Carol Haber's essay and book on mandatory retirement in the nineteenth century and William Graebner's book on the history of retirement.[1] Though their studies largely agree as to the underlying data, Graebner stresses the economic determination of cultural concepts, while Haber emphasizes the convergence of economic factors and "beliefs, motives and decisions."[2] These studies will be reviewed in some detail, at the expense of repetition of material already discussed, because they are the only two book-length examinations of the historical data.

Culture and Economics

In early America, though the concept of retirement was known, retirement was not a normal event. If involuntary retirement did occur, it was commonly for individually determined reasons, not because of age. Certainly there was no custom to retire just because some fixed age had been reached. For farmers, final retirement in the sense of gift or sale of the homestead to a son was common for men in their late sixties, but most men died before they reached that age.[3]

Mandatory retirement is thus a novel practice, invented in the last century. The demand by a wide variety of companies that workers automatically retire at some specific, predetermined age first arose in the late nineteenth century. Even as late as 1890, only about one-quarter of all aged workers considered themselves permanently unemployed. The first businesses to adopt pension programs were connected with the railroads. Such a program was first proposed by the American Express Company in 1875 and first put into full operation by the Baltimore and Ohio Railroad in 1884.[4]

Haber identifies several causal factors for the rise of mandatory retirement. First, these firms had to deal with the most powerful unions. Their pensions programs were, in part, paternalistic welfare programs intended to pacify disruptive employees. Additionally, since the grant of a pension was discretionary with the employer and required long, uninterrupted, and satisfactory service, the programs gave the employer more power to discipline its workers. Second, she explains the muting of union opposition to forced retirement by its connection with recognition of the seniority system. Even in the current era, she notes, while the AFL-CIO opposes unilateral compulsory retirement, it has accepted this condition when acceptance of a seniority system hinges on it.[5] Unions were attempting to establish seniority systems to limit management favoritism; one cost of seniority for the firm was that cutbacks would leave them with senior, highly paid workers. A mandatory retirement policy put a limit on the cost of the seniority policy and was demanded by employers as a *quid pro quo*.

Haber argues, in the third place, that retirement was consistent with a late-nineteenth-century tendency to categorize human capabilities. "The popular view of aging held that, by the very process of becoming old, the aged employee necessarily had to be less productive than his younger counterpart. . . . The industrial pace, all agreed, used up the laborer, leaving him at sixty-five little more than a shell of his youthful self."[6] Similarly, managers of charities assumed that the old did not need to, and could not, work. Proposed factory acts to protect worker health would have prohibited labor by the elderly along with banning child labor and restricting the working hours of women. Efficiency experts appeared and similarly advocated retirement as part of the new concern with efficiency. (Neither Haber nor other scholars, however, have been able to find any actual studies by the experts advocating retirement that demonstrated in fact the correlation of age and efficiency.)[7] According to this view of the aged employee, the pension system thus served to rid the firm of its overpaid and underproductive members. They would be replaced by young workers, who would be paid less and produce more, increasing overall profits.

In sum, Haber's account is that in the late nineteenth century, in part because of widespread immigration, there was an oversupply of labor in a rapidly industrializing society. She describes the reactions of several groups. Members of benevolent societies who administered charity began to allot work to the younger poor; it was not considered necessary that the old engage in work. Efficiency experts and others propounded theories that younger workers would be more efficient, leading industrialists to adopt forced retirement to enhance productivity. Industrialists set up pension systems as part of efforts to achieve a stable and disciplined work force; the age-based pension helped legitimate mandatory retirement. Unions sought seniority systems, which increased wage costs; firms sought mandatory retirement to limit such costs. In these several ways, "the restrictions that limited the employment of the elderly were consciously devised in an attempt to regulate the labor market."[8]

Haber's explanation of the rise of mandatory retirement thus turns largely on substantive rationality: the aged were thought to be used up as workers. Process rationality reasons do not seem to her to have been important: no special attention was paid to difficulties of individualized measurement. Indeed, employers do not seem even to have bothered with studies of the average productivity of different age groups. As a matter of intertemporal choice and preference for routinization, workers (through their unions) seemed to accept mandatory retirement as a trade-off for seniority protection. Haber also emphasizes that age-work policies were instances of the growing bureaucratization of society, the tendency of large institutions to proceed by generalization and rule rather than by individualized determination.[9]

The pension system, though in principle separable, was historically associated with mandatory retirement; it gave mandatory retirement enhanced legitimacy. The pension aspect of the retirement system also had the systemically rational value of giving management more control over workers and encouraging long and faithful service. Little or no evidence of overt intergroup competition is reported, though a background of labor surplus is assumed. Though younger workers obtained jobs, the initiative in the job transfer remained with the employers, motivated by conceptions of relative efficiency. Mandatory retirement was also associated with a seniority system; employers would grant union demands for the latter only together with the former. On the whole, the package may have benefited older workers at the expense of younger ones, though the package would obviously benefit those aged 55–65 at the expense of those aged 65–75. Union decisions to acquiesce to such packages may thus be an instance of intertemporal choice on the part of older workers.

Haber's study reveals no evidence of prejudice (hostility or ambivalent attitudes) but only of stereotype (mistaken factual beliefs). Though she characterizes mandatory retirement as a practice that "broadly discriminated against the old and, in effect, created a legitimately segregated class in modern society,"[10] in the end she rejects the hypothesis of intergenerational attitudes.

The Economic Basis of Ideas

We now turn to Graebner's account. Though Graebner's underlying data largely agree with Haber, he writes in a different tradition. Graebner regards beliefs and attitudes as a superstructure reflecting fundamental economic factors; he specifically rejects the notion that mandatory retirement was based on a culturally widespread mistake.[11] Instead, age-work ideas reflect the economic relationships in a capitalistic society; those relationships have fostered a variety of ideas—in the New Deal, the right to a pension; in the 1950s, the ideal of a golden period of retirement; in recent years, the concept of age discrimination. It is Graebner's thesis that the driving forces behind retirement policy are macroeconomic. In recession or periods of declining activity in specific industries there is reduced demand for labor, and workers have to be excluded from the work force.[12] When international competition or new labor practices threaten profits, productivity must be increased and less efficient workers must be excluded. When the dependency ratio worsens, the economy requires more persons to be retained in the work force as producers.

Against such macroeconomic contexts, Graebner seeks to explain why older workers are singled out for differential treatment through policies unfavorably reshaping the position of the elderly and the middle-aged in the work force. (That phenomenon is referred to by Graebner as "age discrimination," but he is not completely happy about the choice of term because it carries the implication of "unenlightened prejudice" as its cause.[13] This study uses the more neutral term "age-work effect" for the phenomenon.) In Graebner's view, the most important causal factor for such age-work policies as mandatory retirement is the employer's conscious concern with efficiency, an explanation in terms of substantive rationality. Mandatory retirement policies first became prevalent in the half-century or so before the Great Depression; economy or efficiency was among the most important causes.[14] Introduction of the shorter workday in that period led employers to try to maintain profits by increasing productivity.[15] Similarly, establishment of minimum wage rules under the Depression-era NRA led to the firing of workers who were believed to be less efficient.[16] Moreover, new technology was thought to require speedier and more adaptable workers. The idea that use of younger workers would increase productivity was spread by economists, scientists, physicians, and experts in the new scientific management.[17] The perceived physical problems of older workers were the most important concern, as shown in a survey by the National Association of Manufacturers.[18] Employers' concern with output and cost-effectiveness led them to turn to presumably more productive and less highly paid younger employees.[19]

Various employers regarded different groups of workers—sometimes the older ones, sometimes the younger—as troublemakers. This preference is a cohort and period effect, varying from time to time. To the extent that passivity or union affiliation is considered a job-relevant characteristic, employer attention to these factors is another instance of substantive rationality.

As to process rationality, Graebner notes the irony that mandatory retirement was established out of a concern for efficiency and that the retreat from it is now demanded in the name of a new efficiency. Graebner quotes recent calls for individualized decision making on retirement to replace generalizations—demands that business make the necessary hard, objective decisions rather than take the "lazy man's way out."[20] These calls for a new efficiency, he suggests, derive from the perceived national need for increased productivity. They suggest that the previous use of generalizations was not only "lazy" but also inefficient. Faced with the need to improve efficiency, businesses find that the use of age-based generalizations has been counterproductive all along.

According to Graebner, a preference for routinization, for depersonalized processes, was among the most important causes of retirement policies.[21] In small firms, the personal relations of employers and employees made involuntary retirement uncomfortable and infrequent. In larger firms where workers were organized into large, manageable units, involuntary retirement systems were practical. Even in the larger firms, though, outright dismissal would have made labor-management relations unfriendly, and retirement was thus preferable. Compared with individual selection for discharge, a retirement system was impersonal and egalitarian. Preferences against individualized decision making on retirement were expressed by business leaders on grounds of administrative costs, the difficulties of accurate assessment, and the consequent disagreements between employers and management.[22]

Graebner also emphasizes employer concern with the influence of the retirement system on overall national political stability, through its effect on the general unemployment rate. It would have been useful had he further explicated why individual employers take into account the effects of their decisions on national rates.

Interesting information is supplied on the hypothesis that mandatory retirement is a result of intergroup competition between young and older workers. Graebner concludes that in industries with a surplus of workers, retirement provided labor with a way to accelerate the transfer of work from one generation to another. Unions favored pensions because they opened up jobs; retirement was unemployment relief, removing older men to make room for the younger.[23] For example, in the 1930s the railroad unions supported retirement because they preferred having the elderly on a pension to putting the young out of work on unemployment insurance.[24] In the recession periods of 1948–49 and 1957–58, unions accepted negotiated mandatory retirement clauses on the lead of their younger workers.[25] The AFL-CIO argued in the 1970s that unions should be allowed to bargain for mandatory retirement: where unemployment is a problem they wanted to be free to decide to allocate work from older to younger workers, since the older workers could receive Social Security payments.[26] Presumably, if unions affirmatively desired mandatory retirement (rather than merely tolerating it), employers might accept the practice as part of the trade-offs in bargaining.

Nevertheless, Graebner offers some evidence inconsistent with the intergroup competition model. Young Chicago teachers, for example, were opposed to the new system of pension plans, and retirement was more popular in unions with high concentration of older workers.[27]

The data just cited are relevant also to the model of intertemporal choice and suggest lack of support for that explanation. Individuals deciding to support or oppose age-work policies apparently did not do so on the basis of long-term calculations of their own life plans and did not deal with the present elderly as proxies for their own older selves. Instead they looked to their short-term, immediate interests. Younger workers are said to have frequently opposed pension systems, seeing it as an immediate cost and an unlikely benefit, and often not finding value in the mandatory retirement feature. Employed elderly workers who wished to retire saw a near-term benefit in pensions, saw no problems in the mandatory retirement feature, and thus often supported retirement systems. Older workers who wished to continue working, apparently a minority, opposed it because of the mandatory feature.

Intergenerational attitudes are considered and largely rejected as a causal factor by Graebner. He quotes modern commentators who say that stereotypes or prejudice have produced a phenomenon of age discrimination comparable to race or gender discrimination.[28] Senator Harrison Williams spoke of the unemployed elderly as "the victims of pervasive, ill-founded myths. . . . The plain truth is that misconceptions regarding the older worker's own desires and abilities are the sole basis" for not employing them.[29] Graebner disagrees with an explanation in terms of age discrimination, though he credits the earlier ideas of the unproductivity of the elderly as being influential, and points out that writers in science, management, and medicine formerly taught that the aged were less productive.[30] His data support the hypothesis that both accurate generalizations and stereotyping (adverse and inaccurate factual generalizations) have influenced age-work decisions.

Modern gerontology teaches that rigid generalizations on the unproductivity of the aged are unwarranted,[31] but Graebner concludes that the current movement against mandatory retirement[32] is independent of new scientific data and derives instead from recognition of macroeconomic realities such as the dependency ratio and international competition.

In addition to factual stereotyping, other hypotheses of intergenerational attitudes include those of unconscious ambivalence and overt emotional prejudice against the elderly or middle-aged. Graebner does not report data supporting these hypotheses, and his historical research has great value on the nonexistence of overt prejudice. His methods are not designed, however, to reveal data on unconscious processes, and thus his failure to find evidence of unconscious ambivalence toward the elderly is not dispositive.

Graebner's history suggests a multifaceted explanation of mandatory retirement. Retirement was thought to replace inefficient workers with efficient ones, and expensive personnel with cheaper ones; it was associated with tenure and seniority; its use replaced personal relationships in business, one aspect of the larger process of depersonalization; it was a form of unemployment relief, shifting jobs from one group to another; it reflected the cultural norm of efficiency in a return to judging performance by standards.[33] His conclusions are consistent with explanations in terms of rationality and intergroup competition.

Graebner's historical account has been discussed to this point in terms of the typology of models of age-work policies. The following paragraphs review his analysis in terms of the extent to which it explains the several characteristics of age-work policies which a satisfactory age-work theory should explain.[34] As a full-length history of retirement, Graebner's work deserves careful analysis, and such an analysis can also serve as an example of the use of the list of characteristics as testing points for age-work theories.

Graebner emphasizes that the causes of expansions and contractions of the total labor force are macroeconomic factors like depressions and declines in specific industries; he emphasizes concern with the dependency ratio. His explanations of the age-work effect parallel those of the other authors discussed above. Older workers are singled out because they are believed less cost-effective, because many wish to stop working and some are willing to give up jobs to younger workers, and because the availability of Social Security and pension benefits makes unemployment for the elderly seem less harsh to both unions and employers.

The choice of one date for retirement rather than another is caused by the macroeconomic forces that affect labor demand and supply. Generalized policies are adopted for several reasons of process rationality and routinization. Individualized decisions are difficult and costly to make and may cause labor-management conflict. Moreover, larger businesses generally prefer routinized, impersonal policies.

Union support of age-work policies is conceived of as a reallocation of work in times of job scarcity. Older workers are thought to be better off living on pensions and Social Security than the young would be on unemployment insurance. Young workers usually have more influence than older ones in some union decisions, for unexplained reasons. In other situations, it is older workers who support retirement systems both because of altruism and because of perceived self-interest. There is support for the hypothesis that some of the elderly altruistically are willing to yield scarce jobs to the young.[35] Other older workers simply wish to stop working.

Larger companies are more likely than smaller ones to have mandatory retirement policies because of a general preference for rationalization; they are free to adopt such policies because of the absence of personal ties between employer and employee. Ebbs and flows in mandatory retirement policies are traced to macroeconomic forces which affect the demand for and supply of labor. Graebner does not explain the trends in behavior in terms of changed ideas about the elderly, rejecting the causal role of attitudes, but it is unclear that his rejection is established from the evidence.

There are several phenomena in age-work policy for which Graebner's analysis does not provide explanation. These are the nondiscretionary characteristic of *automatic* policies, the related phenomena of absence of renegotiation and nonhiring, and the variations in policies among similar firms. Graebner does not separately address these practices, which involve employers' use of strong forms of generalized policies permitting no individualization. The only reasons for these phenomena suggested by his analysis are the preferences of larger firms for uniform rules (preferences that are not analyzed) and the current criticism that firms are "lazy."[36] These phenomena will now be addressed.

Renegotiation of individual wages and job assignment, like individualized retention of existing workers, is an alternative to a nondiscretionary policy. In the general case, Graebner does not explain the nonrenegotiation phenomenon. In the case of those older workers whose work product is less than the minimum wage, it is obviously the governmental rule that prevents renegotiation. Graebner reports one occurrence thus explained, when the imposition of minimum wages under the NRA led employers to lay off older workers believed to be inefficient enough so as not to be worth that wage.[37] Yet Graebner does not cite an NRA rule allowing retention of the infirm elderly on subminimum pay: "Persons who are limited in their earning power through physical or mental defect, age, or other infirmities, may be employed on light duty below the minimum wage . . . and for longer hours . . . , if the employer obtains . . . a certificate authorizing the employment of such defectives in such manner."[38]

As to automatic compelled retirement, Graebner notes process rationality reasons: there are administrative costs associated with individualized evaluations, they are difficult to make, and retirement based thereon may generate ill-will. These observations do not, however, sufficiently explain employers' self-denying failure to use individualized decisions to retain satisfactory employees when an evaluation system is already in place, as is often the case.

Graebner does cite one example illustrating reasons for a specific automatic retirement rule—that contained in the first Railroad Retirement Act of 1934.[39] When that act was passed, the railroads objected to its mandatory retirement provisions as depriving them of valuable employees. In *Railroad Retirement Board v. Alton R.R.,* the Supreme Court agreed that a policy forcing older workers to retire "irrespective of their fitness to labor" was not a reasonable means toward the supposed statutory purpose of promoting safety.[40] If that statute is seen as in fact a work-sharing measure, a manifestation of intergroup competition rather than of substantive and process rationality, such a competitive purpose explains the nondiscretionary features. Younger workers presumably want older, efficient workers to retire even more than they wish older, inefficient workers to do so. Apart from his discussion of this statute, however, Graebner's analysis does not trace the adoption of automatic policies; his study thus leaves that phenomenon largely unexplained.

Failure to employ older workers is the application of a nondiscretionary policy to new hires. While Graebner depicts the seriousness of the problem of middle-aged persons seeking work, he gives no explanation of why an employer would apply a flat bar in spite of evidence of individual capability. The association of compulsory retirement with pension plans is also not sufficiently explicated. And Graebner does not explain why firms with similar economic positions vary in their age-work policies.

11 • The Labor Department's Theories

The Age Discrimination in Employment Studies

In 1981 the U.S. Department of Labor submitted to Congress, as required by the 1978 ADEA Amendments, the *Interim Report to Congress on Age Discrimination in Employment Act Studies.* That document, prepared by Malcolm H. Morrison and Betty H. Roberts on the basis of several contracted research studies, contains the main data, and there is also a shorter and more popularly written final report.[1] The *Studies* contain at least four different explanations of mandatory retirement, without making their interrelation or relative importance clear; Morrison himself also published later under his own name an explanation of mandatory retirement that differs from those of the governmental report.[2]

A section at the beginning of Part 2 of the *Studies* attempted "to document the reasons for the existence of mandatory retirement policies."[3] These studies took several approaches to that task: an account of the historical development of mandatory retirement policies, including a discussion of the impact of the unions; a statement of employer and employee rationales for mandatory retirement; and a discussion of recent economic explanations of mandatory retirement. Still another theory of the "function of mandatory retirement" began Part 1 of the *Studies,* drawing on survey data as well as upon a theoretical *backstop model.*

Historical Account

The Labor Department's historical narrative is not clear because causal claims are not explicit, the account is given out of chronological sequence, and accounts with different emphases appear in different passages.[4] It can be restated as follows.

The emergence of age discrimination in employment in the United States can be traced to the late nineteenth century.[5] In the next period, from 1900 to 1930, the chief labor benefits obtained by workers were not pension plans supporting retirement, but reduction in hours of work at younger ages. When Social Security was enacted in 1935, one of its clearly understood purposes was to encourage older workers to leave the labor force by providing an economic base for retirement and thus to provide more jobs for younger workers. Social Security established retirement as an expectation. It is "generally agreed" that the age limit of 65 was an arbitrary choice. Yet, once chosen as the minimum age for receipt of Social Security retirement benefits, it became the actuarial basis for private plans. Widespread adoption of formal pension plans did not begin, however, until the 1940s, and the primary purpose then was to speed up retirement by executives. Only thereafter did pension coverage gradually spread to the general mass of employees. Not until after World War II did reductions in work at older ages surpass overall reductions in working hours as a major labor supply trend.

This historical account suggests different causes for mandatory retirement practices at different periods: age discrimination in the late nineteenth century, the provision of jobs for younger workers during the Depression of the 1930s, encouraging executives to retire in the 1940s. One of the intriguing aspects of this account is that it highlights the period after World War II—half a century after the first mandatory retirement plans—as the time of the major growth of such plans.

A number of authorities have suggested the importance of unions in bringing about the acceptance of mandatory retirement; the Labor Department's report gives special consideration to the position of the unions.

Prior to the 1930s, unions were strongly opposed to compulsory retirement and fought to keep such provisions out of contracts. During the Depression of the 1930s, union policy softened "to at least tolerate, if not advocate" mandatory retirement.[6] In the late 1940s and early '50s, with economic conditions improved, unions tried to extend the working years of older members by raising the age of mandatory retirement or attempting to abolish such policies. McConnell and Corson found, however, that as of their study in 1956, unions had done little to protect older applicants from age discrimination in hiring.[7]

Historically, unions' attitudes toward mandatory retirement have been ambivalent, "an ambivalence reflective of union attitudes toward older workers generally." While unions "rarely supported mandatory retirement actively," "tacit acceptance" seems to have played some role in its continuance, especially when mandatory retirement was part of a pension plan.[8] It is "generally agreed" that the effect of collective bargaining on the presence of mandatory retirement in pension plans "followed no obvious trend." A Labor Department study in 1957–58 of 100 collective bargaining agreements on pension plans found that one-half included compulsory retirement provisions and the other half did not. Other studies found that unionization had "no significant effect" on the presence of mandatory retirement provisions in pension plans. "Although the degree of unionization was highly related to pension coverage, it was not a factor in the incidence of mandatory retirement."[9]

Rationales

The historical rationales for the causes of mandatory retirement are set out in the *Age Discrimination in Employment Studies* and can be analyzed in terms of the models used in this work.[10] Employers' reasons for mandatory retirement focused on rationality. In terms of substantive rationality, employers believed that productivity decline was commensurate with increasing age. The substantive rationality reason was combined with several process rationality explanations supporting age-based generalizations as more desirable than measuring productivity of individual workers. Age-based generalizations were desirable because use of generalizations is cheaper; it is administratively easier and thus more practical; the bureaucratization of large companies requires simple, uniform rules; and the procedure is impersonal and impartial, avoiding charges of favoritism or bias, and thus lessening conflicts which may result in appeals.

Employees came to accept mandatory retirement at age 65, according to the Labor Department, because the strong economic incentives of Social Security and employer pension plans, as well as social expectations, led to the attitude that age 65 marked a natural boundary between work and retirement. Moreover, a compulsory system, by avoiding performance evaluations, made retirement in dignity possible. It also encouraged financial and psychological planning for retirement.

Another reason was given for using retirement rather than renegotiation: decreased productivity could not be reflected in changed wages or employment conditions because union rules created an inflexibility in wages, work rules, and seniority.

A reason for mandatory retirement shared by both workers and firms was that it made possible promotion of younger workers, which was hindered by seniority practices. (This systemic rationality explanation, mentioned in passing in the historical Part 2 of the *Studies,* is elevated to prime position in the explanation given in the same report's Part 1, to be discussed in a moment.)

Economic Explanations

The *Age Discrimination in Employment Studies* also presented recent economic explanations of mandatory retirement as "another point of view" alongside the historical explanation. The report does not make clear the relationship between the two kinds of explanations. It may be that one set of explanations is incorrect: perhaps the historical explanation merely presents rationalizations, the beliefs held by firms and workers, while the economic explanation depicts the true underlying causes of which the beliefs are a mere superstructure. Alternatively, the historical explanation may present beliefs that were indeed the operative causes of age-work practices, while the economic explanation may be an attempt to find some functional justification for those practices.

The economic explanation is presented in the following form. Mandatory retirement practices are a consequence of free-market contracts. Workers freely choose to take and stay in jobs subject to such practices. In giving up free choice with respect to retirement age, workers must receive some benefit not otherwise forthcoming. That benefit is a share in the advantages that come from long-term employment contracts.

Workers prefer long-term contracts because there are search and set-up costs in beginning a new job, and it is optimal to spread these costs over as long a job relationship as possible. A different way of putting the point, not suggested by the Labor Department, would take into account that past search and set-up expenses are already sunk costs. A worker anticipates the monetary and psychological costs of moving to a new job, and decides that the move is worthwhile considering not only the increased compensation per year but also the expected duration of the new job, long enough to make the transition costs worthwhile.

Firms prefer long-term contracts to reduce search and hiring costs and to gain maximum return from investment in human capital. Withholding part of the reward for present work gives the firm some leverage in ensuring satisfactory work by the employer. The Labor Department seems here to make the assumption that the promise of a future carrot may sometimes induce more or better work than payment of the present carrot. And while the report does not make the point, the sharing with employees of some of the increased profits to the firm accruing from these strategies would then give employees a reason to accept the practices.

The Labor Department concludes that a pattern of data gives relative support to the long-term contract theory of mandatory retirement: high-productivity industries and high-wage jobs are linked with age-work policies. While jobs with physical requirements are more likely to have pension coverage, they are less likely to have mandatory retirement rules. Since physical strength and speed are qualities particularly likely to decline with age, this datum points away from substantive rationality explanations of mandatory retirement. Unionization, the department says again at this point in its discussion, is not a factor in mandatory retirement practices.[11]

The economic explanations set out by the Labor Department show why long-term employment relationships may be preferred but do not explain why they would be terminated by age-based mandatory retirement. A further diffi-culty with the economic explanation is recognized by the *Age Discrimination in Employment Studies:* the economic theories do not explain the puzzle of the universal use of age 65 as the termination point in such contracts.

A possible explanation has already been suggested for use of age 65 as retirement age in the long-term contract perspective. If costs are associated with use of a variety of mandatory retirement ages and if many workers retire voluntarily when eligible for social security and private pension, then there is a reason to set the mandatory retirement age at the typical voluntary retire-ment age.[12]

Moreover, working past the date of pension eligibility often reduces the value of the pension, thus effectively reducing the wage rate. This pension characteristic might encourage older employees to reduce their work if they were retained. Presumably there are potential gains from establishing an op-timal retirement age for individuals or firms rather than using the arbitrary age of 65, but apparently such gains are too small to overcome the effects of the pension rules. This last argument "weakens the importance of the long-term contract theories," according to the Labor Department.[13]

If retirement at a certain time is desirable to the firm, the Labor Depart-ment points out, it can be accomplished without mandatory retirement. The pension-plan eligibility age by itself can encourage retirement, and in addi-tion, a nonneutral pension plan can encourage retirement at a desired age by making the lifetime value of the benefits different depending on the timing of retirement. Without benefit of the studies done after 1981, the Labor Depart-ment concluded that nonneutral plans probably have "at least as much" to do with inducing retirement as mandatory retirement rules.[14]

Survey of Employers

A different discussion of the causes of age-work practices is set ouf at the beginning of Part 1 of the *Studies.* Using a theory of "the function of man-datory retirement," the report relied in part on data derived from the National Survey of Employee and Employer Responses to the 1978 ADEA Amend-ments, a study that include 6,000 randomly selected workers aged 40–60, all covered by the ADEA, and their 5,800 employers.

Observing that mandatory retirement practices are far from universal, this theory uses as its starting point the same kind of test used in this work: the functions of mandatory retirement can be inferred in part by comparing firms that used the practice and firms that did not. The only distinction between the two groups of firms the Labor Department analysis mentions here is size:

larger firms used age-work practices more than smaller firms. This analysis did not try to draw conclusions from other common distinctions between firms with and firms without mandatory retirement, such as type of industry. A second strategy of the study was a direct one: personnel officers of firms were asked their reasons for using mandatory retirement. All firms, but particularly large firms, put greatest emphasis on assuring promotional opportunities for younger workers, what I call systemic rationality. The promotion rationale was stronger than the often mentioned rationale of retiring unproductive workers, what I call substantive rationality.[15] A survey of firms retaining mandatory retirement after 1978 showed that they "believed age limits were more important as a way to assure promotional opportunities than as a way to remove unproductive workers. The larger the firm the relatively more important providing opportunities for younger workers became."[16]

The relative unimportance of substantive rationality as an explanation for mandatory retirement was supported by other findings. Company personnel officers were surveyed by the Labor Department about performance evaluations. The survey served as one test of the process rationality theory that mandatory retirement practices serve in place of performance evaluations as alternative means to protect both firms and workers from the risks of age-related decline in productivity. Survey results showed that firms using mandatory retirement practices were *more* likely than other firms to use formal performance evaluations. This finding is inconsistent with the process rationality theory that age-based generalizations are needed because direct performance evaluations are unavailable or undesirable. Among the 1,376 employees of firms that did not use mandatory retirement, 66.6 percent of the workers were subject to formal performance evaluation, and 33.4 percent were not evaluated. Among the 1,687 employees of firms that did use mandatory retirement, 87.6 percent were subjected to formal performance evaluation, while only 12.4 percent were not.[17]

Beyond that datum, after mandatory retirement was restricted by the ADEA, the firms with mandatory retirement reported they were no more likely to make their performance evaluations more strict. "These results suggest that age limits did not act primarily as a substitute for formal performance evaluations" but "more often operate in conjunction."[18]

Another set of findings also tends to show that systemic rationality is more important than substantive rationality as a cause of mandatory retirement practices. Personnel officers were asked about the anticipated effect on the cost of labor if a large number of older workers were to postpone their retirement to age 70. Personnel officers of firms with retirement firms, compared to those without, were twice as likely to expect an impact on the number of vacancies, and the larger the firm the more nearly unanimous the response.

Yet firms with retirement policies were four times as likely to believe that cost of labor would *decrease* should many older workers postpone retirement: firms employing 21 percent of manufacturing workers—34 percent for the largest firms, those over 30,000 employees—so believed. This was the same group of firms most likely to retain an age limit and offer financial inducements for early voluntary retirement; these steps presumably were taken for some reason other than controlling labor costs.

A number of other practices beside mandatory retirement are used by the same firms towards the goal of producing sufficient vacancies through retirement. Among these other practices are a relatively early age of pension entitlement and such financial incentives for early retirement as the continuation of health insurance. Firms with mandatory retirement plans were found to be significantly more likely to offer such early retirement incentives than firms without such plans. The incentives were regarded as quite effective: among employees covered by a mandatory retirement rule, 79 percent were in occupations where employees retired on average by age 65. (No data are reported in this analysis comparing retirement and nonretirement firms for average voluntary retirement date by occupation.) The reason financial incentives are generally effective, the argument goes, is that most employees make their retirement decision on the basis of a "target income": they want to retire as early as they can, provided that they will have an adequate retirement income.

This explanation of the function of mandatory retirement is labeled a *backstop model,* since it argues that firms use the practice as a backstop to other incentives intended to produce early voluntary retirement. The overall purpose of the retirement practices and related inducements is assumed to be what I call systematic rationality.

The backstop role of mandatory retirement, according to the Labor Department's analysis, is significant: a mandatory retirement rule does have an effect on voluntary retirement. Survey data were used to estimate the impact of mandatory retirement practices on individual voluntary retirement, using a model of the determinants of an individual's planned retirement age that included the person's demographic characteristics, financial circumstances, current pension and Social Security entitlements, and some characteristics of the firm's pension plan. The results were consistent with the target-income model of retirement. For most men, an age-65 retirement rule does not influence the wish to retire early. But for about 20 percent of the individuals, such a rule influences their planned voluntary retirement date by a year or two.[19]

The picture suggested by these findings is that of mature firms, large and growing slowly, which seek to keep workers for their entire careers. Given the absence of rapid firm growth, in a hierarchical structure the firm uses promotional ladders to retain its labor force; promotion thus involves movement into already-existing slots. Mandatory retirement, the conclusion goes, is a policy to help assure that enough slots will be open, and a trickle-down effect will multiply the promotional possibilities created by each retirement. While the Labor Department's analysis actually speaks in terms of predictability of vacancies, the number of openings seems more important.

Why does a firm adopt the systemic rationality goal? The analysis suggests that firms seek to retain long-term employees either because they believe workers must have a substantial amount of firm-specific human capital or because of the firm's management philosophy. Since invested capital depreciates and time is necessary before returns are produced, some firms view the better treatment of younger workers as economically rational. Retiring older workers to increase promotional opportunities is seen as a way of keeping younger workers, as part of a system where the typical worker will stay until the usual retirement age.

The Labor Department analysis did not try to relate these findings to the conclusions reached in other sections of the same report, such as the historical reasons for the growth of mandatory retirement practice. Nor did the analysis consider problems with the explanation in terms of systemic rationality—e.g., Why is a forced retirement policy applied to low-level employees whose departure does not open up promotions? Why is there not use of the alternative policy of required transfer from high-level positions? Why is not a quality judgment, rather than an age-based rule, used to create the desired number of vacancies among senior employees?

The Labor Department's analysis also suggests quite a different explanation for age-work policies. If there is a reduced demand for labor, "the choice may then be between an older worker retiring with partial compensation, and a younger worker's keeping [*sic,* but should be "losing"] a job. In that event, the socially preferable alternative has been to retire the older worker."[20] The analysis does not explain why it is "socially preferable" that the older rather than the younger worker be removed from the work force on reduced income.

III • The Studies of Aging

Part 2 dealt with studies on the causes of mandatory retirement. But many explanations of mandatory retirement involve external factual assumptions: they are analyzed in this Part 3. Here, I review studies of older persons' physical and mental characteristics, considering the hypothesis that mandatory retirement can be explained by certain characteristics inherent in aging (that it "inevitably wears us all down"). A key section, Chapter 13, surveys the research on the productivity of older workers. If older workers are indeed less productive, that fact would support rationality explanations for the practice of mandatory retirement and imply the normative justification of the practice as economically rational. But if the research does not support the hypothesis of diminished productivity of older workers, the topic of attitudes toward them, discussed in Chapters 15 and 16, assumes special significance. Does research reveal a general antipathy toward the elderly or, in the absence of such antipathy, is there nevertheless a common erroneous belief among management—a stereotype—that older workers have diminished productivity? In the last two chapters, I use theories drawn from psychoanalysis and cognitive psychology to explore the possibility of unconscious ambivalence or general cognitive error. Perhaps different normative judgments and government interventions are appropriate for emotional bias than for factual error.

12 • What Is Aging?

"Aging—almost by definition—inevitably wears us all down," is the Supreme Court's commonsense theory.[1] This chapter considers whether that proposition is accurate by briefly reviewing current biological definitions of aging.

Etiology

Why do we grow old? This question has only recently been the object of concerted biological research considering the aging of the organism, its systems, and the cells of which it is constituted. Aging, or senesence, occurs in all multicellular animals except possibly those that grow throughout their lives; animals that grow to a fixed size and then stop growing eventually die and may be said to have a stage of senesence.[2] A number of theories of the etiology of aging have been proposed; the theories are largely conflicting, though scientists note that theories on the causes of aging are increasingly seen as overlapping. The dominant theories may be divided into intrinsic and extrinsic theories.

Among intrinsic theories the earliest theory holds that aging is pleiotropic—a harmful by-product of necessary functions. Either there is an active degradation occurring through the same forces responsible for life, or metabolic "garbage" builds up and eventually chokes off the processes that created it.[3] Several researchers report evidence that aging is inherent in body cells.[4] A different set of theories hold that aging results from the progressive accumulation of the results of genetic errors, which gradually impair the cells' ability to function.[5] The error theories have a counterpart in repair theories: while cells have an ability to repair certain types of damage to their DNA, this ability is not constant, and it may be that aging occurs through a gradual failure of the cells' ability to correct errors.[6] Some recent research indicates that the set of genes regulating the immune system affects the rate of aging. This same set also influences DNA repair, the production of free radical scavengers, and other process, so perhaps several theories of aging can be grouped under this "genetic umbrella."[7] One of the more philosophically interesting possibilities is that aging occurs more or less "on purpose" as an active program of debilitation.[8] There may even exist special aging genes, directing the organism toward its death.[9]

A variety of extrinsic theories also are extant. The principal opposition to intrinsic theories revolves around the observation that cells, like the organisms they compose, are subject to an array of abuses, which eventually take their toll. The external forces may conveniently be divided into those of wear and those of tear. The principal wear factor is the accumulation of wastes mentioned previously.[10] There are several varieties of tear factors. Free radicals (atoms or molecules with an unpaired electron such as those of oxygen) are highly destructive to other molecules; the molecules thus destroyed may build up in cells, useless but unmetabolized.[11] Temperature shock can also impair cell functioning, possibly by impairing the action of enzymes, the proteins that carry out the work of a cell.[12]

Physiological changes within the body of an organism may detrimentally affect the functioning of cells. The immune system may lose its effectiveness, thus leaving the organism more susceptible to damage caused by other organisms.[13] The immune system may also lose the all-important ability to distinguish "self" from "nonself," causing the body to fight a battle with its own tissue.[14] Finally, it has been suggested that changes in the endocrine system (which exercises hormonal control over the development and functioning of the body) may cause it either to lose control or to exercise too much control.[15]

Emerging concensus indicates that there is no single cause of aging; efforts to isolate one causal factor have largely faltered.[16] In any given individual, one or another cause of aging may be dominant, or several may act in concert. The impairment of organs varies among individuals. Whatever the answer, scientists agree it is likely to be complex.[17]

No agreement on the mutability of the rate of aging exists either. Some scientists believe that the life span of the human species is fixed at about the age of the longest-lived individuals now known;[18] others believe that dramatic changes in maximum life span are possible.[19]

Changes

The characteristics of aging are many and varied and can be measured with varying degrees of accuracy. Some of the better-described changes are physiological, and many of these are quite marked. For example, the speed of transmission of nervous impulses, the basal metabolic rate, and the amount of standard cell water decrease approximately 20 percent from age 30 to age 90. Cardiac index, kidney filtration rates, and lung capacity have been reported to drop 30 to 60 percent over the same time. Biologically, there seems no question that there is an effect; metabolic rate and the ability to respond to biological stresses are reduced.[20]

There is no simple relationship between the typical process of biological aging and the changes in functioning that also, confusingly, may be called "aging." Six patterns of change in older persons were identified in the Baltimore Longitudinal Study of Aging.[21] In addition to "precipitous" old-age declines and steady declines despite the absence of disease, there also are declines resulting only from illnesses that themselves are associated with age. Other biological changes are actually reflections of cultural changes. Moreover, there is also a pattern of stability and a final pattern of compensatory changes that mitigate declines. Thus, absent illness and culturally induced dependency, many older persons will not exhibit serious declines.

Some functions do not change, or change only a small amount: the Baltimore study reports that personality is relatively unchanging. Many cognitive functions undergo substantial decline only after age 70, and even then the effects are mitigated to an extent by compensatory changes, as we shall see in the next chapter. These changes may be hidden or highlighted by period and cohort effects; variation from year to year or generation to generation are not truly age-related factors.[22] As mentioned earlier, some scientists believe that there need be no extended period of decrease in functioning, and that functioning at close to maximum potential can be maintained until just before death.[23]

While the many changes of aging are quite measurable, one is left with the question of whether the changes affect older persons so as significantly to reduce their productivity. This question is explored in the next chapter.

13 • The Productivity of the Older Worker

In addition to studies on the biological nature of aging, there is a body of research dealing directly with the factual predicate of substantive rationality theories: the desirability of older persons as workers. The age-work policies that assumed older workers have lower productivity were originally adopted without any formal studies having been conducted.[1] In the years since initiation of those policies, however, there have been a number of studies. They have been summarized in several reviews of the research literature, including the 1983 book by Doering, Rhodes and Schuster, *The Aging Worker;* the 1983 second edition of Woodruff and Birren's *Aging: Scientific Perspectives and Social Issues;* and a chapter by Davies and Sparrow in the 1985 work *Aging and Human Performance.*[2]

Summary of Conclusions

While the evidence on the age-performance relationship is mixed, the widely held negative belief about older worker performance does not have strong support in the evidence.[3] The studies performed so far have failed to show a great overall decline in job performance at about typical retirement age.

Age as a Proxy of Performance

The 1965 report of the Secretary of Labor, *The Older American Worker,* concluded (in italics) that "the competence and work performance of older workers are, by any general measure, at least equal to those of younger workers." It added that a comprehensive review of available medical and psychological evidence revealed "no support" for the broad age lines which have been drawn on the basis of claimed physical requirements. "To the contrary," the research "has established that there is a wide range of individual physical ability regardless of age."[4] Riley and Foner, summarizing what was known about the elderly in 1968, reached similar conclusions.[5] The Federal Republic of Germany concluded in 1974 that "it should be made clear that older workers do not as a rule suffer from lower performance."[6] The 1978 Report of the Senate Human Resources Committee that led to the ADEA Amendments of that year made similar factual findings.[7]

The Aging Worker concluded, "The performance of older workers is not necessarily either better or worse than that of the younger workers."[8] Older workers in general are more desirable employees than younger workers in several respects: they are less likely to leave the firm, have lower rates of avoidable absence, and have lower rates of overall absence. The job performance of older workers may be positively influenced by such factors as level of motivation, self-reliance, recognition, work-place climate, experience, and job demands. Older workers consistently express greater overall satisfaction and report higher levels of internal work motivation and job involvement. In general, the research indicates that their job attitudes and work behaviors are congruent with effective organizational functioning.[9]

A 1980 survey of the research concluded that "despite age-related changes, research studies over the last 30 years have documented that chronological age is not inevitably correlated with productive capability."[10] Workers between 60 and 75 "are functionally able to produce in many different occupations," and some "may actually excel because of their judgment, experience, and safety of performance."[11] Other studies agree that older workers, on the average, have been reported to "hold their own" against younger workers in a number of different occupations,[12] and that in some job fields in which experience is at a premium, older workers perform better than younger ones.[13]

Variability

A number of studies have reported that the average difference in performance between age groups is typically significantly less than the variation within each age group, rendering age a poor proxy for productivity.[14] For example, studies of comparative job performance, by age, of office workers and of production workers found relatively little variation in average performance among age groups, but considerable variation among individuals within any one age group.[15] Indeed, many older workers' performance is at a level at least equal to the average level of their juniors.[16]

Welford concluded in 1958 that "though performance slows somewhat with age, variation among individuals increases with age."[17] Thus age is an even poorer predictor as persons grow older: "Chronological age by itself cannot be used as an accurate indicator of either the health status or the physical capacity of older workers."[18] Indeed, some writers suggest that chronological age is useless as an indicator of physiological decline. At whatever age, chronological age turns out to be a poor predictor of performance in a wide range of activities.[19]

Theoretical Capacities versus Actual Performance

Age can lessen particular physical or mental capacities,[20] but there are several reasons those changes in theoretical capacities may not render actual job performance unacceptable. Those capacities may not be required for job performance. Or the capacity required for the job may be sufficiently below the capacities initially possessed by the worker so that, even after decline, the worker is still able to perform satisfactorily. A wide range of occupational requirements fall well below the usual range of personal capacities subject to these requirements.

There is an increasing capacity of the human system to compensate for diminishing abilities. The workers may be able to make up for decline by adopting new strategies (*unconscious optimization*) like listening more carefully or by using new aids like eyeglasses.[21] Even though speed and strength may decline, studies show that the overall rate of output can be maintained by older workers, even when doing heavy work, if the moment-to-moment pace of production is established by the individual.[22]

The job as well as the surrounding environment can be redesigned to accommodate the changing abilities of older workers. For example, lighting can be improved, noise levels reduced, the pacing of tasks slowed, the design of machine tools improved to make the tools simpler to use, and buffer items introduced on conveyor belts so that there is flexibility in timing to offset momentary slowness.[23] Steps can also be taken to reduce exposure to such environmental stresses as dusty or polluted air and very high temperatures, and to minimize such causes of difficulty as postural load and movement and muscular load.[24] As OECD reports document, other aspects of the job can also be redefined or reassigned to meet the needs of the older worker.[25]

Matching the individual to the task is also important, as shown by the OECD studies. A worker unable to perform a previous task may still be able to perform another one, for example by giving up the heaviest labor. With seniority older workers can avoid the tasks that embarrass their particular capabilities. They can move into jobs that make use of their experience and to self-paced tasks that avoid the repetitive machine-paced tasks for which the older nervous system is not ideally suited. From the forties onward workers drift away from machine-paced tasks that demand speed into self-paced tasks.[26]

The Nuffield Foundation studies point to increasing differences of individual performance with advance in age. Yet, they show, at the same time, an increasing capacity of the human system to compensate for diminishing abilities and a wide range of occupational requirements which fall well below the usual range of personal capacities subject to these requirements. "The scientific findings, if they were to be translated into hiring policies, would clearly rule out policies based on rigid age limits." [27]

The generalizations given above are derived from two bodies of research which will now be considered separately: one on overall job performance and the other on traits and behaviors that contribute to job performance—including intelligence, work behaviors, and other specific physical or mental traits.

Job Performance

A number of surveys of managers over the last half century report favorable evaluation of older workers; these are discussed in Chapter 15, dealing with attitudes toward the elderly. There is also a body of empirical research concerning overall job performance. Waldman and Avolio performed a meta-analysis of thirteen studies and found some strong evidence of a positive correlation between *improvements* in performance and increase in age. Summarizing twenty-eight studies over the last thirty years on the relationship between age and performance, they found that the research does not support any consistent generalization on the relationship between age and performance.[28] Eleven studies on various occupations showed no statistically significant relationship between age and job performance. Four studies showed that some older workers' performance was better in terms of output level, accuracy, and steadiness of work output. Seven studies showed an inverted-U relationship between age and performance for scholars, engineers, and scientists, and nine other studies showed performance declining with age, generally reporting "slight" or "slow" decreases at ages 45, 50, 55, or 65. Eight other studies were summed up as "inconclusive."

A study of over 3,000 male and female industrial workers aged 18 through 76, in positions ranging from unskilled labor to lower executive levels, reported that performance-appraisal ratings were not related to age.[29] A study of 1,525 insurance agents found no relationship between age and productivity.[30] Research on almost a thousand men aged 16 through 76, holding skilled, unskilled, and clerical positions, reported that mean efficiency evaluations showed little change up to age 45.[31] Another study dealt with 6,000 workers, mostly women, whose ages ranged from below 25 through about 65 and who were incentive office workers in five federal agencies and twenty-one private companies. Output differences among age groups was essentially insignificant, but considerable variation existed within age groups. Older workers were more accurate and capable of steadier output; only in two fields, footwear and furniture manufacturing, did workers over 65 show declines.[32] Another researcher studying garment workers found that for a speed job (sewing-matching operator) older workers earned less at piece rates; for skill jobs (examiners and materials handlers) older workers earned more.[33]

A large-scale study by the U.S. Department of Labor using production records found that in several industries average performance of 65-year-olds was somewhat below peak levels: for example, in men's footwear (17% below), household furniture (14%), post office mail sorting (8%).[34] A study in two large department stores found that performance improved with age and experience, peaking in the early fifties.[35] While a study of professional engineers suggests that their knowledge base may become obsolete, with each age group above 30 obtaining lower average job-performance ratings than the next younger age group in 1968,[36] there are also several studies of scholarly production over the lifetime which generally show continued production peaking after middle age.[37]

In general, research on overall job performance shows slight decline for older workers in some positions, but not the major and general declines assumed in the conventional wisdom on the elderly.

Specific Traits

Besides this research on overall job performance, there is also research on specific traits of older workers. In some occupations, it is not feasible to measure the individual job performance of the older worker. Thus, productivity is sometimes a function of the team rather than of the individual. For such jobs the useful question may be whether the relevant measurable specific capacities or traits of the older worker decline below an acceptable range. For example, deep coal is mined by teams and individual productivity is unmeasurable; relevant traits like strength can, however, be easily measured. In addition, it is not feasible to have a system of evaluations of actual performance in crisis situations. For crisis-related jobs assessments of specific traits such as intellectual functioning and job-related knowledge may have to be substituted. Since decline in one ability is not necessarily accompanied by decline in others, employers must choose carefully the abilities they wish to evaluate.[38]

Here, we shall review briefly the research on age-related decline in specific work behaviors, abilities, and skills. The Department of Labor's 1965 report concluded that "so far as the allegedly key issue of physical capability is concerned, a comprehensive review of available medical and psychological evidences reveals no support for the broad age lines which have been drawn on the basis of claimed physical requirements. To the contrary. The basic research in the field of aging has established that there is a wide range of individual physical ability regardless of age."[39] Other summaries of the literature are collected in recent volumes edited by Birren and Schaie, Poon, Woodruff and Birren, and Charness.[40]

Work Behaviors

One group of studies deals with the relation of age to "withdrawal behavior": employee turnover, absenteeism, and accident rates. Common sense would predict that older workers will be with the firm for a shorter period than younger workers. To the contrary, studies show that older workers are less likely than younger ones to leave the firm, probably because of higher overall job satisfaction as well as the expected difficulty of finding work elsewhere.

Older males generally have lower rates of avoidable accidents than younger ones, reflecting attendance motivation and attitude toward work. In some instances they do have higher rates of unavoidable absence, due to chronic illness and longer recovery periods after injury.[41] And once injured, they take longer to recuperate; they are also more likely to have fatal accidents or to suffer a permanent disability.

Intelligence

Krauss contends that "considerable evidence has been gathered to demonstrate that age-related changes in intellectual functioning appear later in life than had been previously thought, that such changes occur differently across abilities, and that the rate of change is different for different individuals."[42] Some individuals do show a strong age-related decrement, others show little or no change with age, and a few individuals show increases in abilities across the entire life span.[43] Moreover, the age-related changes in intellectual functioning vary greatly, and many old persons perform at a much higher level than most people younger than they.[44]

Newton, Lazarus, and Weinberg discuss the long-held popular belief that intellectual ability declines with age after maturity is reached and recognize that many studies appear to support this belief. They point out, nevertheless, that these studies do not account for cohort effects: the fact that a succeeding cohort may score higher does not demonstrate decline in any given cohort, but may be a result of better education. Moreover, a number of external variables may well affect the results reported. Increased incidence of ill health, the approach of death, and personality variables could all mask the true relationship of traits and age. Newton and his associates emphasize the importance of not jumping to conclusions and summarize the research as showing that the correlation between intelligence and age is not high.[45]

Schaie examined the longitudinal data and concluded that, within a given cohort, the peak on the verbal meanings test is at age 55 and that "even at age 70 the estimated performance is still of higher ability than it would have been at age 25."[46] There is very little change in intellectual function for an individual throughout adulthood except for abilities where speed or reaction time is very important.[47] Like Newton and his colleagues, Schaie also notes that there are important cohort effects as distinguished from age effects: it is not that the intellectual abilities and skills of healthy old people have declined; rather, it is that in certain respects the young of today function at a higher level than those young fifty years ago.[48] We may observe, although Schaie does not, that some employers then have cause to regard younger workers as likely in general to exhibit better intellectual skills than older ones.

A different cohort effect leads to the conclusion that retirement policies should change over time. James Birren has summarized a Swedish longitudinal study that followed three successive cohorts of individuals at age 70 in Gothenburg. Each cohort was healthier than the previous ones: successive waves of individuals arriving at age 70 are likely to be in better health and have higher capacities for work performance. "By the turn of the century we might have more older persons qualified to be employed," Birren concludes.[49] Moreover, the observed "obsolescence can be remedied by retraining,"[50] and the differences in intellectual performance between young and old often are so small as not to make much of a practical difference. "Often such data are simply used as rationalizations to deny the elderly societal roles they could well handle if they were allowed to do so."[51]

Another major finding is that verbal abilities are more likely than nonverbal ones to remain stable with age, or even to rise rather than decline.[52] Birren and associates have reviewed the empirical literature on intellectual abilities of the elderly. They note that while some scholars take seriously the existence of a decline in intellectual functioning with age, a newer viewpoint emphasizes the evidence for stability of functioning among the elderly. "There are considerable data and soundly reasoned arguments on both sides of the issue," they say.[53] Schaie and his colleagues in their review doubted that there is a generalized intellectual deficit in the elderly and concluded that cohort differences are in general of greater magnitude than age changes.[54] Birren and his co-authors conclude that "Schaie's work represents an important beginning, but . . . the absolute quality of the existing studies does not justify simple, unqualified conclusions."[55]

Memory, Speed, and Other Capacities

The majority of laboratory findings on performance of a number of tasks, according to Davies and Sparrows, conclude that performance deteriorates with age in situations placing heavy demands on sensory and perceptual mechanisms, selective attention, working memory, information-processing rate, and so on.[56] The "two behavioral processes most consistently found to decline with age" are speed of behavior and memory.[57] Data also show declines for reaction time, physical strength, and perception.[58] But older people seem to perform at about the same level as younger people in many tasks requiring sustained attention.[59] Extended practice reduces age differences in performance considerably.[60] And when older individuals are highly experienced at the task they are performing, no age differences emerge.[61]

A body of research on aging and memory shows an age-related deficit in long-term memory: older persons are unable to recall as much of the test material as younger persons. Researchers suspect the deficit is in acquisition or retrieval stages rather than in storage.[62] In laboratory studies using word-list memory tasks, differences between older and younger persons are "large and persuasive." But older persons have shown little disadvantage compared to the young in tasks more like the learning and remembering tasks of everyday life, such as remembering sentences and discourse materials.[63] The ability to recall information acquired over the course of life remains approximately constant, though short-term retrieval appears to be more difficult for the elderly.[64] Learning and memory in the context of everyday life has been studied in another line of research including that of Walsh and Baldwin and Waddell and Rogoff.[65] They consider tasks which are significant in the day-to-day lives of older adults, such as comprehension of sentences and retention of prose material. "A common finding from this literature," Birren and associates point out, "is that when individuals are assessed on familiar tasks that have a meaningful context, age differences are smaller than with traditional laboratory tasks, and sometimes are negligible."[66] A recent review of the literature concludes, "It is clear that at the present time we can make few generalizations about learning and memory differences between older and younger adults."[67]

Mental-processor (problem-solving) ability seems to decline with age; flexibility in approaching the problem appears to be the key. The reason for the decreased flexibility is disputed: one explanation is an increase in "perceptual noise" or extraneous stimulation, while another hypothesis points to decreased processing resources.[68]

Decline in speed of behavior may be due to central nervous system change,[69] but may also be a response to lessened activity[70] or to cautiousness. "There remains a continuous discussion of the extent to which an older subject must be slow, wants to be slow or has a set to be slow."[71] Newton, Lazarus, and Weisberg conclude that all aspects of behavior slow with age, perhaps because of the neurological changes known to occur.[72] Birren concludes that for intellectual tasks involving a high-speed component there is age decrement in most individuals rather early, usually in the thirties. There seems to be rather good consensus on this, he says. But "ability tasks that are commonly utilized in everyday life tend to be insensitive to age." [73]

Horn and Cattell concluded that their theory of fluid and crystallized intelligence is particularly applicable to studies relating adult aging to changes in intellectual performance. Fluid intelligence reflects basic intellectual functioning, such as certain types of reasoning and heavily speeded abilities, while crystallized intelligence reflects training, education, and other cultural influences such as knowledge of vocabulary. Horn and Cattell found that fluid intelligence was higher, on average, for younger adults, but that crystallized intelligence was higher, on average, for older adults. (They also noted the possibility that the averages were affected by sharp declines experienced by only a few people.) [74]

The Horn-Cattell view of a decline in fluid ability in later life is to be compared with Schaie's questioning of the "myth of intellectual decline." In the subsequent scholarly debate, it seems that there is agreement that some decline occurs but with variability in the development of different intellectual abilities of older persons depending on the individual, the task, and the situation. [75]

Problems of Research Design

In evaluating the research on the relation of aging to abilities and skills, one must take into account certain methodological problems which suggest that aging may not be the cause of the declines that have been found. [76] These studies have differed in methodology. The research has sampled adult workers from age 25 to age 60 and above; the two largest groups sampled were blue-collar workers and professors. Sample size ranged from 45 to more than 10,000. [77] There is variation between fields (peaking occurs earlier in mathematics) as well as variations between jobs in the same trade. [78] Only a few studies of age in relation to performance included workers over 65, and results for those workers are not always separately reported.

Research on the effects of aging ideally should use a longitudinal design, testing the same subjects at different ages. Yet, much of the research uses cross-sectional designs, testing at one time subjects of different ages: [79] differences that are found may thus stem from cohort effects rather than aging effects, involving potential explanatory variables other than aging. Since the general population has experienced a rising educational level, for example, the cohort now about 65 (born in the 1920s) will have had less education than the cohort now about 50 (born in the late 1930s). Research should also focus on tasks that involve real work situations. It is not always clear whether one can generalize from laboratory experiments to real work situations: the experiments may lack ecological validity. "Older subjects' reductions in experimental cognitive tasks do not necessarily imply that their job performance will drop below 'expected' standards of achievement" for the additional reason that "many individuals are working well within their cognitive capacities." [80]

Finally, even in longitudinal experiments there is dropout of subjects that may skew the finding. [81] Those older persons whose skills deteriorate leave the work force, and a sample of those still working presents an optimistic picture of the whole cohort. [82] (On the other hand, the most skilled may be promoted out of the sample captured by a research design.) Even if research on those still working does not describe the whole age cohort, however, it can support a different kind of finding of great salience to policy issues. The favorable findings about the performance of the group of surviving older workers supports the adequacy of real world systems of weeding out aging workers through self-selection and present methods of evaluation. A rational firm establishing an economically efficient policy on employing 65-year-olds is less interested in the capabilities of 65-year-olds in general than in the capabilities of those who have persisted in the work force. There is reason to believe that individuals who continue to work after 65 are a particularly able subset of the employee population. The skewing problems of the usual research design are thus not necessarily fatal to the usefulness of the results.

14 • Individualized
Determination of Productivity

Some older workers do show decline in some traits and in performance on some jobs, but not all workers in all traits and in all jobs do. There is great variability among older individuals. It is therefore important to consider the factual predicate of process rationality theories: the assumption that individualized determination of productivity is impossible, or at least too expensive. This chapter considers whether it is possible to evaluate the competence of specific workers, obviating the use of age-based generalizations by making individualized determinations of productivity or of appropriate traits.

Feasibility

For some positions, individualized determination has often been regarded as not feasible. Measurement of a worker's output is not easy where production is organized among work groups or the whole factory and the single worker has little control over output.[1] In such situations, though, as already mentioned, the worker's capabilities can be measured instead.

Measurement may also be difficult for low-skill jobs. One study of arbitrators' decisions observed that "in an industry in which semi-skilled jobs predominate . . . , clearly discernible differences in ability among large groups of employees [are] so slight that they do not govern the selection of persons for promotion."[2] In these situations, though individualized determination is not feasible, generalizations about significant differences would also be unsupportable.

The Supreme Court has also noted that it could be difficult to weed out senior officers on a merit basis if, because of stringent up-or-out reviews, surviving personnel "may all be extremely competent."[3] But then presumably there is no substantively rational reason to force any to retire.

Soon after the adoption of the ADEA Amendments of 1978, Ross noted that "a regular system of performance appraisal [was] normal in some companies but spotty or nonexistent in others. It is a safe bet that such formal evaluations will eventually become a commonplace of corporate life."[4] Several writers called for the establishment of formal performance evaluation techniques to make possible reliable decisions on individual performance capabilities.[5] A procedure was proposed by Krauss as an extension of Cronbach's model that would provide testing for the least able and for those holding non-safety-related positions.[6] More extensive testing would be required for those jobs in which safety is a critical factor. "The tests would be selected or constructed to distinguish among individuals to determine who is capable of performing adequately, not who is capable of performing best."[7]

Rowland concluded that it is feasible to use comprehensive tests of job performance as a substitute for age-based generalizations. There should first be an analysis of the functions necessary for a specific job, and then available medical tests should be used to determine whether an individual is fit as to those functions.[8] Similarly, one court analyzed the situation as to age-based rules for law enforcement jobs: "The physical abilities needed to perform law enforcement duties are easily tested. [There are] many simple and inexpensive tests which can easily assess a patrolman's balance, flexibility, agility, speed, power and endurance. If the [employing agency] is genuinely concerned about the well-being of the public and its officers, it can readily evaluate its members and discharge those who cannot perform up to standard."[9]

Performance appraisal processes have been developed for both private and public employees, though those in the field recognize that no appraisal system is perfect or fully objective.[10] There is also specific work on improving job evaluations, testing, and interviews to produce more age-neutral assessment and evaluation methods.[11] Employees' concern about older workers' declining health has led to the development of tests for general physical condition—such as the well-known GULHEMP.[12]

Moreover, "it seems that the older employee is among the first to realize when the job is suffering. Usually the employee will seek voluntary retirement about this time." Thus, the experience of Bankers Life and Casualty was that "when employees can no longer handle their present jobs, we consider them for other more appropriate positions. If there is nothing more suitable we might have to retire the employee. However, it is very rare when this problem comes up."[13] Those older workers who are disabled by illness typically recognize the fact and retire; the unfit who do not retire voluntarily can be identified by their employers and required to retire by an individualized determination. Most of those older workers who wish to stay on are fit. The ADEA permits firms to lay off unproductive or technologically obsolete workers.[14]

One would think individualized determination must be possible: employers for years have promoted some workers and discharged others. The studies on job performance and on relevant traits discussed above all involved testing of large numbers of workers, indicating that in principle employers might be able to use similar testing to make individual judgments. Employers without mandatory retirement rules have decided which older workers to keep on and which to let go. Indeed, the Labor Department called employers' experience

119

with individualized determination of older workers' merits "the strongest indication of the lack of real basis for most age limitations."[15] Employers with mandatory but nonautomatic retirement rules have also long decided when to make exceptions.[16] The use of individualized performance evaluations by the same firms that have mandatory retirement will be discussed in a few pages.

Cost

The costs of evaluation remain to be considered. In theory, evaluation could be so costly that it would be cheaper to throw out the good with the bad. Indeed, one reason seniority is often used as the basis for wage determination is that, by contrast to the conceivably prohibitive cost of determining productivity on a case-by-case basis, it is "a relatively simple concept which lends itself readily to objective measurement."[17]

Yet, it is important to remember the wide variation in individual abilities among workers of the same age and the relatively small variation in average performance from one age group to the next. Age-based generalization is thus a poor method of selecting out weak workers and will simultaneously result in discarding some of the best workers; this method thus suffers from both underprediction and overprediction, what statisticians call both Type I and Type II errors. Methods for individualized determination of productivity do not have to be very accurate to improve on age generalizations, and thus, less expensive tests and ratings may still prove sufficient.

The existence of personnel merit ratings for salary purposes demonstrates that there would be little or no marginal cost in using them for retirement decisions. In addition to firms using performance appraisals, there are also a number of firms that operate systems of individualized determination to examine physical or mental abilities or general competence for a position. These systems are regarded by management as sufficiently accurate to determine appointment, promotion, or retention, and there would be little or no marginal cost in using them also to determine the involuntary retirement issues. It is true that personnel appraisal systems are sometimes criticized in terms of relevance, reliability, and bias; a rater may, or example, make a stereotyped judgment that age must lower job performance. Ratings nevertheless meet these criticisms better than age-based generalizations. Waldman and Avolio, after reviewing thirteen studies on job performance and age, concluded that older workers were assessed more favorably when objective measures of job-related abilities were used for assessment. They recommended job analyses to identify specific mental and physical requirements for workers in a given job, "intrinsic predictors of job performance," that could be assessed. "The arbitrary use of younger age as an employment criterion would unavoidably discriminate unfairly against an older worker whose capacity remains high."[18]

Ignoring Individualized Determinations

As early as 1964, a survey by the Conference Board of "pacesetting" firms found that most used merit ratings, job-oriented performance appraisals, or appraisal of performance in terms of measurable objectives.[19] The Labor Department's *Age Discrimination in Employment Studies* found that 87.6 percent of employees covered by mandatory retirement after the 1978 ADEA Amendments were also subject to formal performance evaluations.[20] Thus, the great majority of firms using mandatory retirement had performance-evaluation systems in place and operating.

Litigated cases provide significant examples of the availability of existing evaluations systems that could be used for retirement decisions. In several important cases where courts approved mandatory retirement policies as constitutional, systems of individual determination of employees' capabilities were operating. In *Murgia* the Supreme Court spoke of age-based generalizations as a method to make sure that state police officers were physically able, yet the police department involved in that case had a system of annual physical examinations that Murgia himself had passed. In *Vance* the Supreme Court stressed that age-based generalizations were means of insuring that State Department officers could meet the demands made of them, yet the Foreign Service had a system of biannual up-or-out reviews. In *Weiss v. Walsh* the District Court approved the use by state education officials of age-based generalizations to insure that a professor would be up to his job. Yet Weiss, who was thus refused appointment to the Albert Schweitzer Chair in Philosophy, had been specifically selected for that appointment by a rigorous search process—in effect determined not merely to meet minimum standards, but to be the most competent available person in the world for the position.

The statistics and these examples show that even organizations that use age-based retirement may themselves already have available systems of individualized determination. The existence of such systems presumably also demonstrates that similar organizations, currently without individual determination systems, would find them feasible. The side-by-side existence of the two systems—individualized determination and mandatory retirement—demonstrates that in these examples either age was not being used as a proxy for productivity or that it was not reasonable to use it as a proxy. There is no reason to think that as a rule age-based generalizations in fact give better measure of individual productivity than does individual measurement or evaluation.

In cases like *Murgia, Vance,* and *Weiss,* if there was some purpose in adopting a retirement rule, it was a reason other than those we have dubbed substantively and process rational. One cannot suppose that age-based retirement was usually adopted because of the supposed psychological and cultural costs of evaluating employees, since almost nine out of ten workers subject to age-work retirement policies were in fact already being evaluated for other purposes.

Safety Situations

In a special category of situations the impracticality of individualized determinations is frequently argued. These situations are illustrated by a few mandatory retirement cases where firms covered by the Age Discrimination in Employment Act have nevertheless been permitted to use age-based generalizations. There have been three key factors in the reasoning by the lower courts in deciding such cases. The jobs affected safety (such as operating an airplane or bus) so that great harm would be caused by failing to exclude unfit employees. Moreover, in those cases a fact-based generalization showed that employing older workers involves a greater danger to customers, owing for example to an increased risk that older pilots will have a heart attack on the job. Furthermore, employers argued that no satisfactory medical or statistical method existed to identify which individuals in the older, at-risk group would experience the problem. Where these factors coexisted, courts applied the ADEA exception allowing an age-based practice when it is a "bona fide occupational qualification." The standard announced for these cases is that an age-based mandatory retirement policy is justified only where it goes to the essence of the business and the firm can demonstrate factually that it is highly impractical to use individual evaluations to show which employees can no longer work safely and efficiently (or else that "all or nearly all" older employees are unfit.)

In the *Western Airlines* case, the Supreme Court applied the ADEA and struck down, by an 8–0 vote, a rule that flight engineers must retire at age 60. The justices unanimously found that Western Airlines had not shown a sufficient "factual basis" demonstrating that individual evaluation is "highly impractical," and that therefore age-based mandatory retirement was not related to a bona fide occupational qualification.[21] Indeed, half the airlines already operated without such an age-based rule.

In the congressional debate on the 1986 amendments, many congressmen raised questions about the suitability of older police and fire fighters, the practicality of individually determining which ones retained their capacities, and the burden on local governments of justifying their policies to the EEOC and the courts. The compromise reached was to exempt these jobs temporarily from the statue uncapping the ADEA's protection and to commission a scientific study.[22]

15 • Attitudes toward the Elderly

The "common-sense" hypothesis about older workers, as a substitute for individualized determination, seems largely unsupported by the data. Mandatory retirement, like many other social policies, largely grows out of widely held beliefs and attitudes which became popular regardless of whether they were true or whether the facts had ever been studied scientifically. Here we shall examine research into the attitudes and beliefs concerning the elderly, exploring what contributes to their wide acceptance of those feelings and judgments.[1]

Ageism

Are the negative beliefs about the elderly a product of prejudice, of ageism? There are some who trace age-work policies to ageism and claim, with Congressman Claude Pepper, that ageism is like sexism and racism.[2] This line of thought uses a model of hostility toward the elderly to explain age-work effects and other age-based differential treatment. *Gerontophobia* and *ageism* have been widely discussed since Robert Butler coined the latter term. Butler summarized in these words what he found to be the widely held images of the elderly:

> An older person thinks and moves slowly. He does not think as he used to or as creatively. He is bound to himself and can no longer change or grow. He can learn neither well nor swiftly and, even if he could, he would not wish to. Tied to his personal traditions and growing conservatism, he dislikes innovations and is not disposed to new ideas. Not only can he not move forward, he often moves backward. He enters a second childhood, caught up in increasing egocentricity and demanding more from his environment than he is willing to give to it. Sometimes he becomes an intensification of himself, a caricature of a lifelong personality. He becomes irritable and cantankerous, yet shallow and enfeebled. He lives in his past; he is behind the times. He is aimless and wandering of mind, reminiscing and garrulous. Indeed, he is a study in decline, the picture of mental and physical failure. He has lost and cannot replace friends, spouse, job, status, power, influence, income. He is often stricken by diseases which, in turn, restrict his movement, his enjoyment of food, the pleasures of well-being. He has lost his desire and capacity for sex. His body shrinks, and so too does the flow of blood

124

to his brain. His mind does not utilize oxygen and sugar at the same rate as formerly. Feeble, uninteresting, he awaits his death, a burden to society, to his family, and to himself.[3]

It is widely believed that gerontological research has documented that these negative stereotypes are common and have contributed to the difficulties of personal and social aging.[4] A well-known study by McTavish in 1971, for example, read the evidence as demonstrating some attitudinal rejection of elderly persons.[5] Bennett and Eckman more boldly concluded in 1973 that "negative views of aging are shared by young and old alike."[6] There is a broad acceptance in gerontology of stigma theory,[7] which assumes that the elderly are the targets of strongly rejecting attitudes.

Indeed, there is a body of evidence for widespread stereotyping of aging and the elderly, much of which is ambivalent or unfavorable, just what is denominated gerontophobia or ageism.[8] One study lists the commonly held stereotypes of the elderly as being that the elderly are unhappy, feel sorry for themselves, reside in institutions, disengage from society, are either sexless or dirty old men (women), are inflexible and set in their ways, and have lessened intelligence, levels of information and knowledge, and productivity.[9]

Some negative beliefs were shown to exist by the most substantial source of information on public beliefs about old age and elderly persons, the 1975 national survey conducted by Louis Harris and Associates for the National Council on Aging.[10] Respondents to the survey associated "most people over 65" with typical activities such as "watching television," "sitting and thinking," "socializing with friends," "sleeping," and "gardening and raising plants." Harris also reported that a majority of adult Americans agreed with the proposition that old people are not very good at getting things done and that they are not very bright and alert. These opinions appear to range across the population, leaping over differences in race, class, occupation, and geographic area.[11]

The mass media both reflect and shape such widely held stereotypes. Thus, research on television shows that it depicts older characters in stereotyped ways—in traditional and also in reverse stereotypes, both types showing older people in unrealistic situations. Perhaps more important, older people appear on television far less frequently than in real life, and older women much less frequently.[12]

Lutsky's review of the literature agreed that a number of specific misconceptions and negative beliefs about the elderly are common and that older persons are usually devalued relative to younger ones. Some research documents that the elderly are viewed as having greater nurturance, dominance, and aggressiveness, and reduced autonomy, effectiveness, retraining potential, and cognitive abilities.[13]

It is often argued, however, that no intolerance toward the elderly exists. For example, the Secretary of Labor's report in *The Older American Worker*

declared that there was "no evidence of prejudice based on dislike or intolerance for the older worker."[14] Instead, age-work practices were based on
"assumptions about the effect of age on [persons'] ability to do a job when
there is in fact no basis for these assumptions."[15] Representative Burke, for
example, argued that disabilities imposed on the aged stem from error rather
than hostility. Unemployment caused by racial discrimination, by contrast,
was thought to be based on feelings about a person entirely unrelated to his
abilities to do a job. Such motives are not the problem for the older job seeker;
age discrimination is based on assumptions that are quite relevant—about the
effects of age on performance.[16]

Moreover, the fact that the aged receive important social benefits is
sometimes taken as demonstrating that they are a favored, not a disliked,
group.[17] Psychoanalytic literature has pointed out that, because children often
have positive unconscious (as well as conscious) emotions toward their grand-
parents, individuals in their adult life often have positive unconscious (as well
as conscious) emotions toward older persons in general.[18]

Ageism toward Older Workers

A separate body of research exists on specific stereotypes about older workers. There is a "widespread belief" that work performance declines as age
increases.[19] Negative attitudes toward older workers have been found in a variety of studies.[20] Tuckman and Lorge's study of psychology graduate students,
for example, found that up to 74 percent agreed that older workers are slow,
require longer and more frequent rest periods, take longer to learn new procedures, look to the past, and are slow to grasp new ideas.[21]

Rosen and Jerdee studied college business students (presumably the
executives of tomorrow) and older realtors. They compared the degree to
which various traits were ascribed to average 30-year-old and 60-year-old
men. In areas pertaining to job stability (such as honesty and reliability) the
older men enjoyed a preference; elders fared consistently worse in the areas of
job performance, capacity, and potential for development.[22] In a related study,
these authors found that college business students playing the role of manager
were significantly more likely to choose to fire or ignore an employee rather
than retrain him if he were described as being old rather than young.[23]

Similarly, the same researchers surveyed 1,570 subscribers to the *Harvard Business Review* asking them to assume a manager's role; half the respondents were asked to make judgments about incidents where the key
worker was described as older, and the other half were presented with exactly

the same incidents but with younger workers. The respondents viewed the older workers as more resistant to change, less motivated to keep up with new technology, less creative, and less capable of handling stressful situations. The study pointed out that "when managers expect a decline in motivation they might make discriminatory decisions that have the effect of lowering motivation and performance among older workers."[24]

Surveys of employment agencies and employers have shown that many of them believe older workers are less productive, frequently absent, hard to please, set in their ways, and involved in more accidents.[25] Britton and Thomas found that employment interviewers view older workers as lower in performance and more difficult to train.[26]

Thus, the belief widely held by gerontologists that ageism is common is supported by a body of data showing that stereotypes about older persons are held both within the general community and within the business environment.

Does Ageism Exist?

There are nevertheless reasons to be cautious in concluding that ageism is common. A 1981 Louis Harris poll found that 90 percent of all adults and two-thirds of all business executives opposed a mandatory retirement age. Some surveys of managers, as contrasted with the experiments just reported, did not find negative attitudes.[27] Several surveys report managers' high opinion of the productivity of older workers. The previously mentioned 1929 survey of several thousand firms in the National Association of Manufacturers said: "A considerable number of companies reported that they preferred older employees . . . while the investigation disclosed no companies which discharged employees when they reached a given age."[28] A 1938 survey of plant-operating executives showed almost no predisposition against older workers based on low productivity,[29] and firms that currently continue to employ personnel in their seventies and eighties find that many older workers perform as well as, if not better than, younger ones. The New England nonpension firms reviewed in the study by Palmer and Brownell generally believed that older workers retained their productivity.[30] This general conclusion has been reached in many studies. (The recent research on actual productivity of older workers was reviewed in Chapter 13.)

There is also a body of research rather consistently showing the extent to which age is overwhelmed by other stimuli as a source of personal perceptions.[31] And Lutsky's review of the literature has criticized the common gerontological conclusions about the prevalence of ageism.[32] Lutsky emphasizes three distinctions: evaluations versus beliefs,[33] absolute versus relative responses, and attitudes toward a period of life (old age) versus attitudes toward a specific cohort currently occupying that period (the elderly).

Lutsky first notes that many accounts of myths held about the elderly cite misinformed rather than rejecting judgments;[34] the relationship between the two types of attitudes remains to be understood. Lutsky's conclusions emphasizing the importance of mistaken factual beliefs about the elderly is consistent with the findings of a different line of research on cognitive error, discussed in Chapter 19.

Lutsky acknowledges that if one looks at ratings of the elderly relative to alternative age periods or age categories, then the attitudinal evaluations would be viewed as negative or negative to mixed.[35] He suggests, however, that we look at the absolute rather than the relative meaning of the responses of those studied: attitudinal evaluations of both elderly persons and old age have consistently been shown to be more positive or neutral than negative, with the predominant evaluations varying from "moderately positive to moderately negative." Lutsky reads the research as showing the absence of a strong negative stereotype of elderly persons and old age. Elderly persons and old age are "infrequently viewed in a strongly negative fashion . . . it is clear that gerontologists cannot assume that negative attitudes are held in general, [or] that these attitudes (both positive and negative) influence behavior."[36]

Lutsky's argument also emphasizes the possibility that negative attitudes have been common toward specific cohorts of older persons but they may not have been held over time toward other cohorts of the elderly, or toward old age. His point is consistent with the finding (which he does not mention) that age-work practices grew up over a few decades, and now have been largely socially rejected in a short time period. Such time-limited, rapidly changing attitudes may have been based on changing current realities or on cultural assumptions rather than on common psychological attitudes toward aging and death. The latter attitudes, as discussed in the next chapter, presumably have deeper roots and change only over generations.

Lutsky's analysis requires some additional comment. He points out that older persons are often rated positive in an absolute sense (that is, above a theoretical midpoint on a rating scale) though negative in a relative sense (that is, lower than younger persons are rated on the same scale.) He does not draw a conclusion, however, that seems apparent: such a relative negative rating could be sufficient to lead to personnel decisions to let older workers go while retaining younger ones.

He also stresses that negative attitudes deal with some traits, not all, and are more likely to be mistaken beliefs than rejecting feelings. He does not ask why negative, mistaken beliefs grow up in the absence of negative feelings.

Especially when such beliefs lead to harmful actions contradicting conscious positive feelings, psychoanalytic experience suggests we at least explore the possibility of repressed, unconscious negative feelings.

Has ageism been demonstrated empirically? And, if so, is it essentially a matter of attitude (prejudice) or beliefs (stereotype)? Overall, these different strands of inquiry show the existence of relatively negative, mistaken factual beliefs about specific cohorts of the elderly. The debate continues over the possible underlying causes of such erroneous stereotypes in more basic psychological attitudes about the elderly, old age, or death. The next two chapters deal with that issue.

16 • Stereotypes and Cognitive Error

Widely held negative stereotypes about the elderly were discussed in the last chapter, and their validity was discussed in Part II. The disparity between stereotype and reality suggests that perhaps we should look to psychology to explain age-work practices. Within this realm, we may inquire as to the relative causal importance of conscious factual beliefs, conscious evaluative attitudes, and unconscious mental function. Two bodies of literature in psychological theory provide rival bases for understanding the persistence of factual stereotypes concerning the elderly: cognitive error is discussed in this chapter, and psychoanalytic theory will be considered in the following chapter.

The literature on cognitive error draws generally on the cognitive tradition in social psychology and involves a number of seminal researchers.[1] Cognitive-error theory calls our attention to a common error in reasoning that may be central to the study of age discrimination in general and mandatory retirement in particular. This error is the practice of satisfying: accepting a partial solution or partial answer because it appears good enough for the purposes at hand and because learning more about the situation would require the expenditure of much more effort. The seriousness of such an error, and indeed whether it is an error at all, depends on the accuracy of the decision made, the cost of further work, and the relation of the cost of further work to the cost of a mistaken decision. The process rationality explanations discussed above assume that personnel decisions based on age are accurate enough and the cost of individualized determination too great. By contrast, the cognitive error explanation suggests that these conclusions may rest on a common human mistake in reasoning.

A useful entry to this body of work is Nisbett and Ross's book, *Human Inference,*[2] which deals with how ordinary people frequently use erroneous strategies of inference to come to know the social and physical world. As is explained by this theory, people generally use certain preexisting systems of schematized and abstracted knowledge—beliefs, theories, propositions, and schemes—as a way to understand the external world. These "knowledge structures" are useful shorthand guides, but they are sometimes wrong.

Nisbett and Ross use these concepts to offer an explanation for ethnic prejudice which is of so general a nature that, while it does not specifically address the elderly, presumably is applicable to beliefs and attitudes concerning them.[3] Their explanation treats (emotion-laden) "prejudice" and (factual) "stereotype" as equivalent terms,[4] and finds that stereotypes exist for almost every category of people. They assume, "Surely it is simpler and more reasonable to look at mechanisms which might apply equally well to both affect-laden and affect-free stereotypes."[5] Individuals first learn stereotypes by hearing of them from others. Thereafter, stereotypes survive because "people may quite reasonably presume that the culture which has provided them so economically with so many facts is right in this case." Or more accurately perhaps, people may not examine the original basis for their stereotypes any more than they scrutinize other culturally transmitted beliefs.[6] People are also likely to give exclusive, or at least disproportionate, weight to whatever data does support the stereotype, and the stereotype is likely to enjoy at least a kernel of fact. In addition to the availability of at least some confirming cases, biased assimilation of evidence and similar psychological mechanisms are also likely to be at work. Thus, Nisbett and Ross argue that "there is no compelling reason to assume that ethnic stereotypes differ in their origin or nature from any other kinds of stereotypes, or for that matter from any other beliefs, good or bad."[7] Their analysis of ethnic prejudice would seem to apply *a fortiori* to ageist stereotypes and to support the conclusion that mistaken factual beliefs, rather than hostile emotions, are involved in negative attitudes toward the elderly.

Cognitive theory asserts that people also generally use certain *judgmental heuristics*.[8] That theory will be here applied to age-work issues. Two rules heuristics in particular have been identified as important by Kahneman and Tversky: the "representativeness heuristic" and the "availability heuristic." The term "representativeness heuristic" refers to a style of thinking well known to the law: faced with a new item, people generally consider the extent to which its features are typical of some preestablished conceptual category rather than another. They then think of the item as a member of the category to which it was assigned. The relevance of this concept to age-based generalizations is clear: a worker may be thought of as a member of the class of older workers, rather than as an individual with his or her own specific capacities. The problem is that to the extent the label is not fully appropriate, unthinking use of it may lead to inaccurate results.

The second term, *availability heuristic*, refers to a style of thought in which judgments that some events occurred are based on the extent to which they are readily "available" in memory. The problem here is that the things most available in memory may not be the best guides to the real world. Thus, isolated gaffes in functioning by elderly persons may be remembered more readily than more common, but unremarkable, competent functioning. An intuitive strategy Nisbett and Ross find to be often—and erroneously—used by ordinary people is the weighting of data most heavily if it is most vivid and salient. Data that is vivid to the senses or freighted with emotion will be taken into account more than pallid data. Again, emotion-based observation of error may be more heavily weighted than pallid satisfactory work, and again the problem is that the most vivid data may not be the most reliable evidence.

Taken together, these theories about knowledge structures and judgmental heuristics refer to cognitive, perceptual, and inferential errors that are widely made in the thinking of ordinary people.

Nisbett and Ross's basic argument on prejudice, it should be noted, is a shifting of the burden of proof: they regard their argument as parsimonious, explaining prejudice as an instance of normal mental process, and see no reason to adopt any other. They do not offer any explanation of how it comes about that the culture changes its beliefs about older workers, or of why the distribution of ageist cultural stereotypes and age-work employer behaviors should reveal certain social patterns. Thus, the characteristics of the phenomenon that we have identified as puzzles are not adequately explained.

Though Nisbett and Ross equate the terms *prejudice* and *stereotype,* the distinction can still be maintained. We may ask whether prejudice (affect-laden attitudes) or stereotypes (beliefs) empirically are more salient as causal factors in bringing about age-work practices. Nisbett and Ross's version of the question is to ask whether prejudice is a matter of "hearts or minds." They question "whether the right organ has been singled out for blame" by others and suggest we look to the mind—that is, to factually based beliefs. The cognitive-error theory looks to nonmotivated, nonemotional, nonspecific general fallacies in typical human reasoning as the casual factors at work.

Cognitive-error theory is to be contrasted with other theories—such as the psychoanalytic—which seek the salient causal factors in motivated, affect-laden, specific attitudes toward the subject at hand (though the attitudes may be relatively inaccessible to consciousness). These latter theories are discussed in the next chapter.

17 • Prejudice, Ambivalence, and Psychoanalysis

Psychoanalytic Viewpoints

Psychoanalytic thinking suggests some hypotheses through which to understand age-work practices. It teaches that feelings are often ambivalent; psychoanalysts have found that hostility may exist notwithstanding simultaneous overt positive feelings.[1] Furthermore, attitudes may be relatively inaccessible to consciousness. Thus, unconscious hostility may coexist with conscious and unconscious respect and benevolence. Persistent beliefs about others' shortcomings in the face of contradictory evidence (for example, ageist stereotypes) combined with harmful behavior (such as adopting age-work policies) may indicate just such unconscious anger. There are several internal conflicts that might generate ambivalence toward the elderly.

One's Family

Support of retired elderly by working middle-aged persons in an intergenerational transfer of income. Such transfers used to be made chiefly within the family; they are now increasingly made between workers and nonworkers through public programs irrespective of family ties.[2] Nevertheless, unconscious intrafamily emotions may still provide the roots of the feelings the middle-aged have about older retired persons. Conflict between the middle-aged and elderly can be conceived of as intergenerational conflict between cohorts of children and parents. We may not regard the aged as proxies for our future selves, as assumed in the intertemporal choice model the Supreme Court implicitly used in *Murgia*. Instead, we may unconsciously regard the aged as representatives of the older people who have been most important to us, our parents. One psychological study, for example, shows a correlation between favorable or unfavorable perception of close elderly relatives, and presence or absence of unfavorable stereotyping of the aged.[3] It is possible that one's unconscious attitudes towards one's own parents are generalized to an attitude toward the older generation through a psychological phenomenon similar to clinical transference.[4]

Current age-related disputes, including legislative and legal issues, may revive internal conflicts buried within each individual. Older persons may be misperceived on the basis of individuals' unconscious attitudes toward parents stemming from childhood. It needs little discussion for one to realize that there are many psychological causes for individuals to feel ambivalence toward the older generation.[5] Among the prior intergenerational conflicts each individual has experienced are Oedipal conflicts involving ambivalent love-hate and both rivalry and identification with the older generation. There are also other conflicts common at other life stages: the infant's conflicts with mother over frustrations, and separation and individuation; the adolescent's rejection of his parents in a shift to peer-group ties; the adult's conflicts over succession to the work and family roles previously held by his parents. Unconscious hostility may be reflected in some, if not all, of the widespread stereotyping of aging and the elderly.

Conflict about Supervising One's Father

Even without assuming unconscious hostility toward the elderly, psychoanalytic thinking suggests another hypothesis that may explain part of the motive for mandatory retirement policies. Managers may have irrational reasons to turn to fixed retirement policies as a way of avoiding individual determination of the value of older workers. A younger man may find it uncomfortable to be the superior of an old man, and even more so to have to evaluate him and tell him it is time to retire. Unconsciously, the manager may feel that the situation represents playing a father's role to one's own father. In the family, the older man represents power and is surrounded by a web of strong emotions. The manager's situation may feel like a role reversal and arouse unconscious conflicts. Even if it is more efficient for middle-aged managers to determine individually which older worker must retire, it is hard to act as an economically rational manager when one's inner forces are stirred up.

One's Own Aging and Death

A supplemental psychoanalytic hypothesis involves attitudes towards one's own aging and death. Several studies have indicated that avoidance of the aged may be a function of one's fear of death, no doubt a widespread anxiety.[6]

Some research, however, has not found a significant relationship between death anxiety and stereotypes about the elderly,[7] nor evidence that those who view the elderly unfavorably think more about death.[8] A clue to reconciling these findings may be Becker's suggestion that while the specter of mortality looms large in the unconscious of each of us, we unknowingly deny our anxiety about death.[9] A study attempting to test a similar hypothesis found a correlation between death anxiety and ageist attitudes. More important, it also found, at least for males, that the *combination* of high anxiety about death and a tendency to use the psychological mechanism of repression was associated with unfavorable stereotyping of the aged.[10] It may be that repressed (i.e., unconscious) death anxiety underlies ageist attitudes. If so, then issues which unconsciously function as surrogates for the issues of death may be most affected by such conflicts.

If there is widespread ambivalence or hostility toward the aged—perhaps unconscious but manifested in conscious stereotypes—one may ask why such a feeling might be particularly influential on age-work issues. The hypothesis concerning feelings towards one family suggests no direct answers, but the hypothesis concerning feelings toward supervising one's father is directly on point. The hypothesis concerning feelings towards one's own aging and death gives another clue. It is possible that in the eyes of many individual employers, retirement—the end of active work life—may symbolically represent death. We may speculate that for an employer to select a particular individual for involuntary retirement may unconsciously feel like selecting someone for death. If many decision makers do indeed have unconscious anger against the elderly, such an overt expression of the antagonism as depriving them of work—symbolically, of life—may come too close for comfort to the unconscious wish. The decision makers may thus unconsciously feel guilty. A less overt expression of the wish may then be sought.

An employer's requirement of retirement thus may function to express an unconscious wish of eliminating the older generations; simultaneously, delegating such decisions to an automatic policy, like a fixed age-point, is a way of avoiding anxiety which is connected with the posited unconscious thoughts. The myth of golden retirement, like the imagery of heavenly afterlife, may also help deny related anxieties.[11] Similarly, we may speculate that the prohibition of mandatory retirement might have the unconscious meaning to a lobbyist or lawmaker of symbolically outlawing, or at least postponing, death.

Parallel Explanations

Irrationality in the Firm

The hypotheses I offer in this chapter are congruent with those explored in a recent volume, *The Irrational Executive: Psychoanalytic Explorations in*

Management, which asserts that "a myth of organizational rationality needs to be reexamined in the context of what is known about the role of the unconscious in human motivation and its impact on decisionmaking."[12] Management theorists should not assume a rational decision maker but should instead take seriously Simon's concept of bounded rationality as characterizing administrative behavior, and its implication that there are limits to individuals' perceptual and information processes.[13] Individual managers bring to work with them their own psychopathology, which may or may not be congruent with their job. The individual's unconscious conflict and intrapsychic defensive behavior may lead thus to "unconscious collusion" by a number of persons in an organization.[14]

A related point is argued by Kevel in *Capitalism and Infancy: Essays on Psychoanalysis and Politics:* that "administrative rationality," in addition to realistic purposes, has an additional psychological purpose as "a defense against the deepest anxieties."[15]

While I have found no studies that specifically focus on the hypothesis of a psychoanalytic interpretation for retirement practices, some reports appear consistent with that theory. Levinson concluded that managers often feel a misdirected concern for employees with long service and therefore fail to confront them about unsatisfactory performance. He also found that intrapsychic conflict arises in a younger man who must exercise authority over an older one; the younger manager may feel guilty and want to appease the senior.[16] Menzies, studying a hospital nursing service, found that individuals used the organization in their own psychological struggle against anxiety, by developing "social structured defense mechanisms." Among the mechanisms she observed were the use of depersonalization or categorization to deny the significance of individuals and to obscure personal responsibility for decisions.[17]

An analogy may be drawn to a provocative article by Bernard Diamond analyzing present-day welfare laws as if they were symptoms of a social neurosis. He noted the intensely ambivalent quality of the social attitudes behind our welfare laws and speculated that the attitudes arose out of the cultural equivalent of infantile conflicts: the society simultaneously loves and hates its poor, dependent, and other "nonpersons." These nonpersons, he argued, symbolically represent the child in a large-scale Oedipal struggle; the potent and socially integrated members of society collectively symbolize the father. "This Leviathan father replicates on the larger social scale, the intensely ambivalent attitudes toward society's children—the various types of nonpersons—that the individual father has towards his own child. The law thus becomes the formal expression of this collective Oedipal neurosis."[18] Diamond's theory has been criticized as speculative and overemphasizing irrationality.[19] Within its own framework, it may also be criticized for speaking as if society could have a "neurosis" rather than speaking of a type of individual widely found within society; furthermore, it treats Oedipal conflict as the sole root of all ambivalence, even though other psychodynamic conflicts may also be at work. Nevertheless, my own speculations, similar to Diamond's, are attempts to state a viable psychoanalytic hypothesis on widespread culturally manifested attitudes to members of an age group.

Unconscious Discrimination

Charles R. Lawrence discusses similar issues in "The Id, The Ego, and Equal Protection: Reckoning with Unconscious Racism." He argues that traditional notions of intent, purpose, or motive do not reflect the "fact" that decisions about racial matters are influenced in large part by factors that can be characterized as neither intentional nor unintentional. Certain outcomes are not self-consciously sought but are still caused by the decision makers under the influence of their beliefs, desires, and wishes.[20]

Lawrence's basic argument is that racist attitudes are largely unconscious, that for the law to deal only with conscious intent ignores much of what we understand about how the human mind works, and that equal protection doctrine aimed at eradicating individuous racial discrimination must therefore recognize racism's "primary source" in unconscious attitudes.

He uses two explanations for the unconscious nature of discriminatory beliefs and ideals. One is the theory he ascribes to cognitive psychology, that the culture transmits beliefs and preference, often by tacit understandings; these beliefs seem to the individual to be part of the rational ordering of her perception of the world. The other explanation is Freudian theory.

Lawrence's article is important and sensitive. Nevertheless, the reader needs to take into account that he largely misunderstands the Freudian theory he attempts to use. For example, he asserts, "First, Freudian theory states that the human mind defends itself against the discomfort of guilt by denying or refusing to recognize those ideas, wishes, and beliefs that conflict with what the individual has learned is good or right."[21] Actually, Freudian theory takes a wider view of psychic defense; it is not just defense against guilt, but defense against anxiety. A person may keep from consciousness ideas that the superego does not condemn but which nevertheless produce the signal of anxiety—for example, thoughts involving one's own aging or death.

It is while we are small children that we develop defense mechanisms about what is most anxiety-producing for us. To a small child, relationships with the parents are likely to be the most affect-laden of experiences. These are the prototypes for relationships between the sexes and relationships between young and old. One would assume that where there is most emotion, there is most room for anxiety, and therefore most likelihood of use of defense mechanisms like repression.

Lawrence also notes the existence of "unconscious sexism."[22] If "sexism is even more deeply embedded in our culture than racism and thus less visible,"[23] he says, and also is less unequivocally regarded as unjustifiable, then sexist attitudes may be repressed less often than racist attitudes and held at an unconscious level less often. Lawrence makes no mention of ageist attitudes, but by his analysis, ageism would be even less subject to repression and less frequently held in the unconscious.[24]

As I understand psychoanalytic theory, Lawrence has the argument backward. Sexist attitudes are, *prima facie*, more likely to be repressed than racist attitudes, because thoughts and feelings about the relationship with the other sex are conflict-ridden experiences for the young child. And if the hypotheses stated above are accurate, ageist attitudes are also likely to be repressed, because the relationship with the older generation is also a highly conflict-ridden experience for the youngster. Thus, in a Freudian theory of repression, unlike Lawrence's theory, commonly held unconscious sexism and unconscious ageism are hypotheses worth considering.

Psychoanalytic Research

The psychoanalytic hypotheses to explain age-work policies could be explored through psychoanalytically oriented research with normal individuals[25] and through research on the manifestations of the culture.[26] One could utilize the analytic techniques of psychohistorians, using sources relevant to evaluation of the emotional processes of decision makers in the present or past. Such techniques would include attempts at psychodynamic interpretation of the imagery and metaphors employed by decision makers. Primary sources would include oral histories, letters, speeches, transcripts of committee deliberations, and other documents already available to historians. Additional sources for an attempt to study shared attitudes would include jokes, folktales, popular songs, and the characters and plots depicted on radio, on television, in the movies, and on the stage, as well as published material in the psychiatric and psychological literature.

The psychoanalytic hypothesis must also be tested against the statistical data. It appears consistent with data suggesting that age stereotyping seems more common when the decision makers are less likely to know the individual aging employees. The small firm is least likely to have a compulsory retirement practice,[27] and the practice is not found among women household service workers.[28] Similarly, supervisors, who are less likely to know the individual aging employees, generally have more unfavorable stereotypes of the aged than do rank-and-file workers.[29] Stereotyped thinking and transference-like effects seem to flourish where they are less challenged by real relationships with older workers. That view of the data is supported by the psychoanalytic finding that restriction of the real relationship (in the extreme, presenting an analytic "blank screen") promotes development of transference phenomena.

Cognitive Theory Contrasted

The difference between the explanations offered by cognitive-error theory and by psychoanalytic theory may be important to the law, because equal protection doctrine often considers motive and differentiates intention from mistake. Psychoanalytic theory gives courts a basis for treating unconscious hostility more like overt hostility and less like innocent mistake of fact, while cognitive error theory seems to suggest the opposite conclusion.

It is therefore important to note the extent to which the cognitive theorists Nisbett and Ross accept the psychoanalytic approach. They quote the prediction of Mandler that cognitive psychologists soon would "rediscover psycho-analytic constructs" under a different terminology.[30] "In our opinion," say Nisbett and Ross, "two of the more basic ideas in our book do amount to a rediscovery of two of the most important ideas with which Freud's name and the psychoanalytic tradition are associated. One of these is the notion that much of mental life is inaccessible to introspection, that is, is unconscious." The other is "Freud's discovery, for it was his, of the enormous importance to mental life of the representativeness heuristic."[31] They also recognize the importance of the psychoanalytic technique of free association as a method of seeking to discover what stands for what in the mental life of a given person. While they note the problem of criteria for validation of interpretations, they recognize psychoanalytic free association and interpretation as a method of reaching a presumptive unconscious meaning of a patient's verbal material: "nothing in current psychological theory or research casts doubt on the validity of such a presumption, and there is much that supports it."[32] They also do not doubt the existence of the mechanism of repression. What Nisbett and Ross basically disagree with is the psychoanalytic viewpoint that "an act must be produced by a correspondent motive."[33] They therefore do not believe that the unconscious meaning of behavior indicates motive states and dispositions that cause it,[34] or that repression of anxiety-producing meanings is a general explanation for the unconscious quality of much mental functioning.

Older workers have been subject to erroneous stereotypes, and these stereotypes have caused them great harm. Cognitive-error theory accounts for

that fact as an instance of general shortcomings of human thought. Psychoanalytic theory, to the contrary, provides hypotheses that would account for the
phenomenon by attitudes specific to the subject matter.

There is nevertheless insufficient research data available to confirm that
psychoanalytic hypotheses explain the age-work phenomenon. I asked Anna
Freud, then already aged but still presiding over the famed Hampstead Child
Study Course and Clinic, for her views about psychoanalytic motivations for
the wish of middle-aged decision makers to adopt mandatory retirement policies. "You do not have to delve so deep," she said to me; "people want to
move up."[35]

Generalization, Stereotype, and Prejudice

Here let me make explicit the distinctions between *generalization, stereotype,*
and *prejudice. Generalization* is defined as the ascription to a person of characteristics without individualized assessment, because of membership in a
category or group thought usually to possess those characteristics. A generalization may be positive, negative, or neutral. It may also be true or false to
varying degrees—that is, category membership may be an adequate or inadequate proxy for the salient characteristic. What Cohn and Thurow call "statistical discrimination" and Posner calls "rational discrimination," what others
call "group discrimination," is negative, accurate generalization.[36]

The term *stereotype* (stereotype proper) is here reserved to mean a negative, *incorrect* generalization. Cognitive-error theorists have concluded that
stereotypes are culturally transmitted theories that persist owing to common
human mistakes in assessing information and drawing inferences. To these
scientists, emotional prejudice derives from stereotypes—erroneous theories
about the factual shortcomings of members of a group. Discrimination, in
their view, is thus not a taste but a way of processing information—not a
matter of hearts but of minds.[37] In the view of these scientists, moreover, contrary to the theories of rational discrimination, use of stereotypes is often not
an efficient strategy but an error.[38] Or, if efficiency must be sought for the use
of stereotypes, it is on a much higher level. The reason an individual fails to
test a stereotype is not that the information costs associated with such testing
are high. Rather, she accepts the stereotype, untested, because of a much
more general decision that culturally transmitted generalizations are usually
accurate and that the costs of retesting *all* such cultural information is too high.

Generalizations and stereotypes, thus defined, are factual ascriptions and
are to be differentiated from *prejudice*—that is, emotional states. Conscious
prejudice is antipathy, hatred, fear, or similar negative affect experienced to-

ward an individual because of his membership in a group or category. A broader definition of *prejudice* would include unconscious hostility, a component of ambivalence, not easily accessible to introspection but detectable through its effects on behavior and mental function.

Legal scholars consider the relationship of findings of prejudice or stereotype to judicial condemnation under the equal protection clause. Intention, or conscious prejudice, is the heart of a finding of discrimination.[39] Only prejudice suffices to come within the legal ban, in the currently accepted view of the constitutional prohibition of discrimination. Similarly, in interpreting a civil rights statute, the Supreme Court held it to apply only when there is a racial or class-based invidious discriminatory animus[40]—in our vocabulary, conscious prejudice. In *Palmer v. Thompson* the Supreme Court had said that a statute's effect, not the legislative motive, is the central equal protection issue.[41] In *Washington v. Davis,* however, the Court dealt with a law that appeared on its face to be racially neutral but had a discriminatory impact upon blacks. The Court held that "proof of a racially discriminatory intent or purpose" is required to show a violation of the equal protection clause.[42]

When a statutory distinction on its face imposes a detriment on a defined group, as with an age-based mandatory retirement law, searches for either "effect" or "purpose" take on a different meaning. We know that the action causes injury to its target and that the detriment is a foreseen result and thus in a sense intended. The decision maker may plead conscious benevolent or economic motives. The psychoanalytic orientation suggests we look beyond the conscious surface for clues as to deeper motives underlying the immediate intent; those clues may reveal hidden prejudice.

Generalizations involving "discrete and insular groups" or those with a "history of purposeful unequal treatment" are treated as suspect by the courts.[43] The courts recognize that laws dealing with those groups may use generalizations as masks for stereotypes, impose unacceptable stigma, or reflect hidden prejudice. But all that may also be true for other groups, such as older workers, which are not "discrete and insular."

Statistical discrimination—which by definition is a fairly accurate generalization, and which may be affect-free—may constitute neither prejudice nor stereotype. If prejudiced intent is the heart of the matter, then use of statistical discrimination with any group should not be sufficient in principle to invoke a strict equal protection scrutiny. Nevertheless, we shall see that the sex discrimination cases discussed below reject such a justification of statistical discrimination justifications; those cases do so as part of a broader rejection of the excuse of "administrative efficiency."

18 • The Psychology of the Work Place

Labor-Management Attitudes

Another set of possible psychological explanations for age-work practices involves attitudes specific to management-labor relations, rather than universal cognitive process or common intergenerational attitudes. The first of these explanations focuses on the personnel process and overlaps the intergenerational model already discussed. Many managers may be unwilling to supervise older workers too closely. The family model involving respect for the elderly may interfere with the work model wherein supervisors are hierarchical superiors.[1] (The family model, supposedly displanted from the factory by cold rationality, continues to return; thus, union members call each other "brother.") The situation of a manager giving orders to older subordinates is salient for psychological reasons, probably arising from the relations of children to their parents. One study showed that French firms took into account the age of the applicant's future superiors as one reason for not hiring older workers, in view of "the fact that many workers are reluctant to give orders to persons older than themselves."[2] Levinson's psychoanalytic study had similar findings.[3] Even managers who believe that a general practice of mandatory retirement is justifiable may still feel uncomfortable about individual dismissals without articulable just cause to dismiss any given individual.

Another explanation is that it may be humiliating to the older worker and embarrassing to the manager to demonstrate that individual cause does exist and drive out the worker in disgrace. Lawrence Friedman, noting that this is a popular argument, summarizes it as "let's not make a scene" and wonders whether its proponents are shedding crocodile tears over the anticipated "distasteful" episodes.[4] Another writer has imagined the scene graphically:

> The premise here is that a large percentage of people really do run out of steam noticeably sometime in their 60s but that it is much nicer not to say so. With mandatory retirement, you can say: "How are we going to get along without you? But you are 65, and you know the rules, and it is a shame." This is much better than telling Joe he can no longer hold down his job and has to leave, and having everybody know why he has to leave.[5]

What this writer overlooks is that it is the manager who may feel that the evasion is "much better," whatever Joe would want. Joe, after all, might be part of that percentage of people who have not run out of steam. For workers who could satisfy job requirements, individualized determination is in their best interests. And other workers may want the option of seeking such a determination, being willing to risk rejection rather than willingly accepting a supposedly stigma-free loss of job.

These feelings of managers may not add up to a justification, in terms of process rationality, for avoiding individualized determination of competence. The psychological costs on managers may nevertheless tip the scale as a causal factor toward adoption of an impersonal fixed rule which allows the manager to disclaim psychologically any responsibility for scrutinizing, evaluating, and discharging individual older workers.

Routinization and a Nonmonitored Atmosphere

Another possible explanation of mandatory retirement involves a different form of psychological meaning to both worker and manager. It is based on the widespread use of routinized decisions involving generalization, not limited to the personnel process. Max Weber wrote of a "formal" rationality in law that is similar to the use of routinized, age-based generalizations for retirement: "law . . . is 'formal' to the extent that in both substantive and procedural matters, only unambiguous general characteristics of the facts of the case are taken into account."[6] Use of age as the basis of decision is formally rational in this sense, since age may be unambiguous; if age is substantively irrelevant, such a formal rationality avoids instances of unfairness only by imposing general unfairness.

Nonmonitored Atmosphere

Formal rules may be valued nevertheless because of their contribution to the mood or "atmosphere" of the workplace. The use of generalization rather than individualized determination for retirement decisions may be compared to the use of a collective contracting mode rather than an individualistic one. Collective contracting is apparently favored by some workers for nonwage reasons:[7] Williamson argued that collective contracting is preferred because the resulting contracting atmosphere is different, and there is less monitoring and metering as to each transaction.[8] For example, the Social Security Administration eliminated individual work-quality standards and production quotas for some workers, keeping records for teams of workers only. "Production and accuracy increased, morale improved, and the use of leave declined."[9] Similarly, some aspects of internal labor markets are valued because they result in a greater sense of justice (absence of whimsy or prejudice).[10] Employees almost always perceive performance appraisals negatively, since their

143

income and self-esteem are at stake.[11] They may have a taste for a retirement policy using generalization just because it contributes to a work atmosphere that deemphasizes individualized determination of competence and emphasizes a feeling of equality.

One study showed that employer disinclination to make individual determinations was frequently given as a reason for a compulsory retirement policy. "Equity" and "uniformity" were often cited as major reasons for such a policy; so was avoiding having "to defend each retirement both to the worker and the union."[12]

Impersonality

It may also be that growth in size and technologically caused reorganization lead to impersonality. Impersonality would not in itself cause age-work practices to be adopted. However, if other reasons for adopting these practices existed (perhaps substantive or systemic rational ones) but were usually inhibited by moral or personal sentiments in favor of retaining older workers, then an increase in impersonality could unleash the underlying reasons. Some support for this hypothesis can be drawn from the finding of a 1958 study that the industries in which older workers find it especially difficult to get jobs are those without a stable work force, where seasonal or temporary work makes it easy to discriminate impersonally.[13]

Size

Employers may also wish to avoid individualized decision making on employee competence because of the difficulties in retaining centralized command control over it. The larger the firm, the more likely it is to have an involuntary retirement policy[14] and age-work hiring policies.[15] Spengler predicted that "there will probably be increasing pressure to throw older workers out of the labor force as control of industry and access to employment becomes still more bureaucratized."[16]

Larger, more bureaucratic companies may also face larger transaction and information costs, leading them to prefer routinized decision making by age-based generalizations. The temporary work industries just mentioned also may find it more difficult to use individualized determinations.

One can, however, challenge the assumption that larger organizations find it more difficult than smaller ones to make individualized determinations of productivity. Large organizations consist of smaller units; the basic working unit may be of comparable size whatever the average size of the organization. Thus, the first- or second-line supervisor, foreman or manager, may have as much information on an individual worker's productivity in a mammoth corporation as does a supervisor in a small concern. Indeed, the larger organization, more than the smaller one, will enjoy economies of scale and be able to afford scientific testing of the individual worker's attributes.

Another challenge to the scenario as to large organizations comes from the finding that, in multiestablishment firms with mandatory retirement policies, the policies were established centrally only a small percentage of the time.[17] Moreover, an indication that such practices may come from below can be found in a survey by the Massachusetts state government in the 1930s. It found that a "large number" of employers explicitly reported that they used no maximum hiring-age limit, but that further investigation showed that "many" of them actually did have such limits, "often without realizing it."[18]

Unions

Unions sometimes support or acquiesce in mandatory retirement. A routinization hypothesis is one potential explanation of the phenomenon. Collective bargaining and mandatory retirement are both instances of dealing with employer-employee relationships by rule rather than by individualized decisions. Perhaps unions may be conceived of as bargaining, not for a mandatory retirement age, but for a uniform retirement age; similarly they often bargain for a seniority system and for a uniform salary for a given job classification and seniority. The union and generalization phenomena then would be subsumed under the heading of routinization. An inclination to make routinized decisions by generalization would also logically deal with many other age-work phenomena—absence of renegotiation, nondiscretionary retirement policies, and nonhiring—as it explains why firms avoid individualized determination of the productivity of older workers. A correlation with size of firm also seems intuitively plausible. In addition, unions may dispute individualized retirements more than decisions which result from generalized policies.[19]

Productivity

Explanations of age-work practices in terms of a preference for routinization are consistent with a controversial body of research suggesting that in many situations a group's work will be more (or at least equally) productive if its members' rewards are egalitarian rather than performance-based. Such a reward system promotes positive attitudes toward the work, feelings of competence among workers, and positive social relationships that are valuable for work requiring coordination and mutual help. This line of thought is set out in Morton Deutsch's book *Distributive Justice: A Social-Psychological Perspective,* which summarizes literature reviews by Johnson, Slavin, and others.[20]

IV • Toward a Theory of Age Discrimination: What Caused Mandatory Retirement?

Parts 2 and 3 have put forth a review and a critique of the major explanations that have been given for the rise and acceptance of the mandatory retirement system. In this part, I make use of that material to move toward a theory of age discrimination. The alternative explanations for age-work practices will be reviewed systematically in terms of the typology of four types of models. I come to conclusions as to the causes of age-work practices and make the judgment that they are generally normatively unacceptable and constitute age discrimination. A fuller ethical and legal analysis of the implications of these conclusions is reserved for another work.

19 • The Four Models

I begin with explanations of the kind I have named "rational" and follow with other explanations that emphasize macroeconomic factors, intertemporal choice, or cultural and psychological factors.

Rationality Models

Mandatory retirement could be a rational profit-maximizing policy in several different ways; one can imagine a number of scenarios in which age is directly relevant to the employer's production process.

Assumptions of Inherent Rationality

Some economic models assume that whatever policy a firm maintains in the face of competition must necessarily be profit-maximizing.[1] Even without such a global assumption, the posit of economic rationality provides a model for explaining the existence of mandatory retirement. Within this model, the key assumption is that mandatory retirement has emerged in response to the interplay of market forces and thus has a rationale in terms of the efficient utilization of human resources. The analysis rests on the belief that the individual parties themselves are best able to determine retirement policy, as part of the total package of compensation and work rules. The collective decision of management and labor can be regarded as an endogenous institutional response to their own trade-offs, thus reflecting the preferences of individual workers as well as of management, and also reflecting the constraints imposed by market pressures and societal pressures expressed through laws and otherwise. The results of the process are assumed to be economically efficient, unless some reason can be given for the existence of a market failure.[2] (The result might nevertheless be regarded as socially undesirable if particular distributional or justice reasons were specified.)

What makes this analysis interesting is the necessity of specifying what particular interests of firms and workers, and which constraints of the market and society, have interacted to bring mandatory retirement into existence. The candidate causes to be considered range from long-term profit maximization to a "taste" for discrimination on the part of employers, workers, or consumers. Let us examine those causes closest to a model of rational employer behavior.

Systemic Rationality

Where retirement of the elderly is thought to have intrinsic value to the system, the term *systemic rationality* may be used. For example, a firm may adopt a retirement policy that requires older persons in top jobs to vacate those positions after limited periods, so as to avoid locking up the firm's leadership posts for long periods.[3] The turnover in work force may be regarded as economically rational even if the younger employees are not intrinsically more able than the older ones they replace, if rotation per se is regarded as economically advantageous. The rotation may be thought to enhance morale, to facilitate the trying of new ideas, to encourage sensitivity to tastes of new cohorts or consumers, or to create incentives for the young by providing promotion opportunities.

Intuitively such explanations seem to have potential validity only for certain types of positions—perhaps management but not assembly-line work. Moreover, unless the ideas of younger workers were considered better than those of the old (which would turn the explanation into one of substantive rationality), a need for fresh blood translates into a need for optimum turnover. There would be a need for involuntary turnover only in the absence of adequate voluntary turnover through resignations, transfers, and voluntary retirement. Explanation would still be required as to why the supposed need for increased turnover could not be met by a variety of other means: by forced transfers to other positions, inducements so that voluntary retirement commonly occurred earlier, or selective merit-based forced retirements. The need for turnover by itself would not justify general age-work policies.

Many personnel managers in the 1980s gave a systemic rationality reason for mandatory retirement, as a backstop to voluntary retirement to make sure that the channels of promotion remained unclogged. This reason cannot have been too weighty, however, because faced with the prospect of losing that personnel tool, they showed little interest in replacing it either with stricter individualized evaluation or with more attractive pension packages to induce more voluntary retirements.[4]

The number of jobs opened up in society by mandatory retirement is not large. As mentioned earlier, one can conclude from calculations by Barker and Clark that the maximum effect of mandatory retirement is to decrease the overall labor-force participation of all men at 65 by about 3.6 percent; compared to the total labor force age 16 and over, the decrease is a small fraction of 1 percent. Thus, the number of middle-aged workers who can move up to positions opened by retirement is also quite small—0.13 percent of the total labor force for men.[5] The total number of promotions would be larger than the number of retirements, however, since openings at the top could create a chain of movement throughout the system.

In any given firm at a given time, historical factors may have created a skewed age profile of employees. If such a firm is top-heavy with elderly senior managers, a mandatory retirement policy will create many vacancies. Nevertheless, forced transfers or inducements to voluntary retirement remain alternatives. The phenomenon of an imbalanced age profile at any given time has nothing to do with old age: a firm may find it has more workers of any given age in a given rank than it would wish and seek to trim the ranks of its teenage messengers or 40-year-old middle managers.

Substantive Rationality

Another common conception of a rational policy of retiring older workers is that age is used as a proxy characteristic for the relevant characteristic of productivity. If it were true that there is a decline in productivity correlated with advancing age, it might be efficient and therefore rational for the employer to use age as a proxy for productivity and to force the retirement of older workers. This scenario requires that older workers be a group with lower productivity than younger workers, in which case we shall say that mandatory retirement can be justified by substantive rationality.

Few explanations of retirement truly focus on age per se. Except for those explanations, the chronological age of a worker—the number of times the earth has circled the sun since the date of birth—is in itself irrelevant, a fact of interest only to astrologers. Chronological age becomes relevant to personnel decisions only when it is treated as a useful proxy for functional age, or rather for functioning—that is, for productivity. Three scenarios may be distinguished:

1. The Overpaid Worker. Even if not regarded as less capable, the aged may be deemed more expensive to employers, because of seniority-based pay scales, increased accident rates, or higher costs for health and life insurance benefits. Even if compensation of the older worker is emphasized rather than productivity, the same conclusion is drawn, that the *compensation-productivity ratio* is less favorable for older than for younger workers.

Some studies, however, question the conclusion that older workers—and particularly older workers in mandatory retirement firms—are overpaid.

2. Human Capital. Even if current productivity is satisfactory, the stream of expected future productivity of the older worker may be thought unsatisfactory. Some argue that forward-looking personnel managers, to be economically efficient, should act on the common-sense belief that the 30-year-old employee will have more growth potential. Moreover, "the case for ageism," according to a *Fortune* column, is that "it's probable that someone who's now 30 will be in the labor force longer than someone who's now 60."[6] Using a human capital analysis, both the depreciation of invested capital and the need for a period of time for that capital to provide returns are potentially economically rational reasons to treat older employees less well than young ones.[7]

There is research, nevertheless, indicating that older workers are likely to remain longer with their firms than are younger workers.

3. Dead Wood.   A third scenario is that in which the aged are regarded as less capable because of a supposed decline in physical or mental ability, in capacity to learn, or in other relevant specific capacities. Alternatively, at any given time the cohort of older workers may be less educated than younger workers, as has been the case in the United States for some time.[8] Many or most older workers may thus be thought to fall below the minimum acceptable level of work.

Employers may believe that at the ages commonly set for mandatory retirement, the productivity of most workers becomes significantly less, or individual productivity losses become significantly more common, either as a more-or-less sudden occurrence or as an accumulation of gradual changes roughly estimated by the retirement age. Half a century ago, the perceived physical problems of workers older than 45–50 and their tendency to slow down were the most important concerns (mentioned over 40% of the time) of the minority of employers who set age limits on new hires, according to a 1929 survey by the National Association of Manufacturers.[9] The complete breakdown of the reasons given in this study appears in Table 19.1

Similarly, physical limitations were the most important reason (mentioned more than one-third of the time) in the study reported in 1965 in *The Older American Worker.*[10] These reasons given by employers for upper age restrictions and for limited hiring of older workers are set out in Table 19.2

Whatever the reality, a belief that the old are poor workers would explain mandatory retirement. In fact, the empirical research suggests that these beliefs are exaggerated. Older persons do not experience physical changes at the same age, and a number of companies have remained profitable despite having many employees in their seventies and eighties.

A supposed factual belief not consistent with reality may be a rationalization or an excuse for bias. Related psychological phenomenon were discussed earlier in chapters on psychoanalysis, cognitive error theory, and attitudes

TABLE 19.1.   1929: Employers' Reasons for Upper Age Restrictions on Hiring of Older Workers

Reason	% of times mentioned
Physical condition of workers	22
Maintain integrity of pension plans: retain work for older workers already employed	21
Tendency of workers to slow down	19
Increased cost of workmen's compensation insurance; liability to injuries; danger to other employees	14
Increased cost of life insurance	11
Total percentage giving reported reasons	87

Source: "Finds Employers Favor No Age Bar," *New York Times*, 21 March 1929, 23.

TABLE 19.2.   1965: Employers' Reasons for Upper Age Restrictions and for Limited Hiring of Older Workers

Reason	% of times mentioned
Physical requirements	34.2
Job requirements	25.1
Company standards	9.1
Promotion from within	8.1
Costs of higher earnings	7.3
Costs and provisions of pension plan	6.7
Lack of skills and experience	6.3
Limited work-life expectancy	5.1
Scarcity of applicants	5.0
Educational requirements	4.2
Lessened adaptability	3.1
Cost and length of training	3.0
Inferior quantity of work	2.3
Slowness in attaining proficiency	2.1
Need for balance of ages	1.7
Undesirable personal characteristics	1.7
Costs and provisions of health insurance	1.4
Costs and provisions of life insurance	1.2
Other	6.8
All reasons	100.0

Source: Sara Leiter, "Hiring Practices, Prejudices, and the Older Worker," *Monthly Labor Review* 88 (August 1965): 969.

toward the elderly. What would cause such unsupported beliefs to arise, change, or diminish? It has not been a universal belief of employers that all older workers are less productive, neither earlier this century nor recently. If some firms but not others based their employment practices on an erroneous factual assumption about the elderly, we would want to know if and how they avoided the discipline of the market.

Process Rationality

Still assuming age per se is not directly relevant to the production process, substantive rationality alone is not generally adequate as a basis for a profit-maximizing decision to mandate retirement. If it were costless to identify the productivity levels of older workers, the use of chronological age as an imperfect proxy could not be efficient. Therefore age-related work policies are rational only when there is also a cost incurred in using individualized determination to identify relevant characteristics. Reliance on the costliness of direct identification of individual workers' productivities provides an explanation for mandatory retirement as process rationality.

Process rationality explanations of mandatory retirement may involve any of several scenarios. They may stress that individualized determination is impossible or claim that it is inefficiently costly. Such a scenario is hard to support in the face of data that almost nine out of ten employees subject to mandatory retirement also were subject to formal performance appraisals. Such explanations may also stress that the use of individual evaluations involves high psychological cost to workers or employers, in which case they overlap the explanations which I discussed in terms of psychology of the work place and preference for routinization. Scenarios that stress the difficulty of explaining individualized determination to workers or their unions resolve into claims either about cost or about psychology.

A different process rationality explanation is that mandatory retirement has value in facilitating planning by both management and workers. Yet adequate planning does not require forced retirement, but only sufficient advance notice. And in large firms experience enables personnel managers to predict voluntary retirement in the aggregate, as they must do anyway to plan for early retirements.

A typical rationality explanation involves both substantive and process reasons for mandatory retirement policies. The relative importance of the two elements justifies identification of separate ideal types of explanations premised on substantive rationality and process rationality. If the hypothesized correlation between age and the productivity characteristic is weak, the cost of directly identifying the productivity characteristic must be great if the mandatory retirement policy is to be efficient—a scenario stressing process rationality. If the hypothesized correlation between age and the productivity characteristic is high, the cost of a more perfect identification of the productivity characteristic could be small and still justify the mandatory retirement policy on efficiency grounds—a scenario stressing substantive rationality.

A comparison may be made to judicial interpretation of the Age Discrimination in Employment Act as permitting age to be used as a proxy for job characteristics only in situations going to the essence of the business where either "substantially all" members of the age group share the target characteristics or most do and individualized determination is "impractical."[11] The first situation involves substantive rationality, and the second emphasizes process rationality.

Unless other assumptions are made, the rationality explanation is inadequate as an explanation of some common characteristics of age-work policies—for example, that some firms' policies are of an automatic type entailing the absence of renegotiation. If the explanation of mandatory retirement were exclusively the decline in productivity with age, one would find it hard to explain why some firms have a fixed rule of absolute discontinuation of employment, rather than retaining the option of changing employment conditions and wages. While it is costly to renegotiate on a case-by-case basis (and conceivably even costly to decide whether or not to renegotiate), an absolute self-denying rule by the employer prevents her from continuing to employ older workers even when their demonstrated continuing productivity, or willingness to take pay cuts, more than compensates for the costs of individual determination. Where a firm has adopted a self-denying policy, the explanation must be sought other than in the firm's substantively rational interest in productive workers. The explanation might lie, for example, in systemic rationality or in union interests in protecting wage rates by limiting the size of the work force.

Other firms do, of course, allow selected workers to continue employment beyond the supposedly mandatory retirement age. In Israel, for example, the government service and the major hospitals do this, and usually employers set up committees to review such requests.[12]

Macroeconomic Models

The models reviewed in the prior section explain mandatory retirement in terms of economically rational decisions by individual firms without overt reference to macroeconomic factors. Another set of rationality explanations emphasizes just those factors. In one version of this explanation, when the overall supply and demand of labor shifts, so does the need for marginal employees such as the elderly.

Another version argues that the need of the economy for productivity undergoes changes in response to international competition and economic conditions. Changed economic conditions could lead to more or less tolerance for less productive older workers, or more or less tolerance for less precise retirement practices. Some economists have concluded that when competition is weak, there is reason to expect greater leeway for departures from profit maximization.[13] Enterprises under such a condition may tolerate extensive organizational slack, involving higher economic inefficiency than one would predict under the theory of profit-maximizing behavior.

A third version of this approach argues that as the ratio in society shifts between the number employed and the number of elderly dependents, this changed dependency ratio permits or requires the employment of fewer or more elderly.

At least for nongovernmental employers, additional analysis is required to specify the link between the macroeconomic context and individual employer decisions. Additional analysis would also be needed to explain the other puzzles of age-work policy, such as the adoption by similar firms of different policies.

Another version of the macroeconomic model explaining age-work effects is that of intergroup competition. One economist, for example, concluded that employers would not have been so ready to part with the elderly as a source of labor supply had there not been women available to take their place.[14] The success of women in this competition was thought to be largely due to their superior education. As to why increased labor supply did not lead to lower wage rates, this analysis implicitly relied on a ratchet-effect argument.

Some use the model of intergroup competition to argue that mandatory retirement opens jobs for women and minorities. A reason cited for opposing the 1978 ADEA Amendments was the predicted negative effect on hiring and promotion of minorities.[15] In general, however, the effect of mandatory retirement on opening jobs is miniscule. As mentioned earlier, the percentage of workers removed from the labor force by mandatory retirement amounts to only a small fraction of 1 percent—0.13 percent of the total labor force for men.[16] Moreover, factors other than mandatory retirement have a far larger impact on work life. Finally, the thesis that older workers are competing for jobs with women and minorities "is the old 'lump of labor' theory, and every economist will tell you that it has no validity," according to economist Walter Galenson.[17]

Intertemporal Choice Models

Still another explanation of mandatory retirement looks to a life-cycle, long-term contract, or intertemporal perspective. The Supreme Court seemed to have accepted such an explanation, among others, in the *Murgia* case. Legal issues in the law of aging do not involve age discrimination, the Court suggested, because we each hope one day to become elderly ourselves: age-work exclusions are explained as directed by "us" against ourselves.[18] Of course, at any given time such actions are taken by one group, the middle-aged, against another, an elderly minority.

A better statement of this model uses as an explanatory concept the idea of choices which arise within each individual's understanding of her own life cycle. A member of the middle-aged majority must balance his own short-term interests in employment against policies protecting his interests in employment later in life. Perhaps work in old age is regarded by most as a "bad" rather than a good; at least, its satisfactions may diminish while the opportunity costs of working increase with the availability of pensions. The individual may then rationally choose *ex ante* to protect the work opportunities of the young and middle-aged and to require the elderly to retire.

As understood in this model, we deal with those presently aged as proxies for our future selves, a mindset which some think to be a sufficient protection against discrimination.[19] Thus, one way to understand age-work issues is that of intertemporal choice: the choice by middle-aged decision makers between immediate and deferred benefits. This model is related to the *life-cycle model* for individual decision, through which economists have begun to study the choice of training, work, and consumption over the course of one's lifetime.[20]

Intertemporal choice might bear on an explanation of even automatic, nondiscretionary mandatory retirement: if almost all workers wanted to retire at a given age, and employers identified with their thinking, conceivably some reasoning based on transaction and information costs might lead to the conclusion that the unusual exception need not be dealt with individually.

We may question to what extent the intertemporal choice model accounts for age-work effects. It is true that in some instances, policymakers do establish retirement policies having in mind their own life cycles—for example, policies for retirement of corporate executives. But in other instances, policymakers explicitly or implicitly exclude themselves from mandatory retirement rules. For example, Congress adopted Civil Service retirement rules but set no limit on ages of members of Congress or committee chairs;[21] Supreme Court justices upholding governmental mandatory retirement themselves had life tenure; the retirement rules for bishops were promulgated by popes who excluded themselves.

Another objection to the theory that individual intertemporal choice causes age-work policies is that people often manage even their personal affairs without much caring about their own interests later in life; *a fortiori* they may make decisions about the elderly as a group without considering their future interests as part of the group. Consider the example discussed by the philosopher Derek Parfit in his new book, *Reasons and Persons*. A boy starts to smoke, knowing but hardly caring that this may cause him to suffer greatly fifty years later. This boy does not identify with his future self, Parfit argues. "His attitude towards this future self is in some way like his attitude toward other people, such as the aged parents of his friends."[22] We can draw the conclusion that if people often ignore their future interests on a topic so personal as cancer, they may do so on a less dramatic topic like retirement policy. Parfit's view of the matter is not that people regard the elderly as their own future selves and so take their interests adequately into account—as the intertemporal choice argument has it—but exactly the other way around.

The intertemporal choice theory might remain a possible causal explanation but be weakened as a normative justification. Perhaps people do try to act toward the elderly so as to safeguard their own future interests, but nevertheless frequently undervalue those interests for any of several reasons. First, they may undervalue their own future interests because our usual modes of cognition apply too steep a psychological discount rate to future pains and pleasures. Even if Parfit is wrong and the smoking boy identifies with his future self, he may discount the future too sharply and thus overvalue near-term interests. Second, internal mental dynamics may give dominance, not just to consciously appreciated near-term interests, but to current unconscious forces. One's attitudes towards one's own later self may be saddled with present unconscious attitudes toward parents or aging and death, to an extent that restricts rational planning. Third, people may not act to safeguard their own future interests because they do not know what those interests will be. A middle-aged decision maker imagining herself at age 65 may be wrong as to whether she then will want to retire or want to work, and may not even realize that her current estimate of future interests is problematic.

Cultural and Psychological Models

Intergenerational Justice

Another set of possible causes of mandatory retirement involves attitudes about intergenerational justice: on fair relationships between generations and on how jobs should fairly be rationed. Public-sector employers, if not private ones, have reason to adopt personnel policies on the basis of their presumed overall good for society, not just on the basis of their effect on productivity. Even private-firm managers are likely to be influenced in their personnel policies by beliefs about fairness and proper social behavior.

Some believe that fairness justifies a rationing of jobs on generational lines: this rationing may be conceived either as equalizing benefits by rotating jobs or as equalizing burdens by rotating discharges. Jobs are seen as a scarce resource to be allocated fairly; the aged have already had their chance at work opportunities, which should now be made available to the young, who in turn will be subject to age-work practices when they become old. Especially in periods of high long-term unemployment, it may be thought important to get young people into employment. Employers may try a strategy of reducing the work of existing employees, incorporating mandatory retirement policies alongside reduction of average work-week.

There is a cultural expectation that those above normal retirement age have a diminished moral duty to work and a diminished moral claim on jobs. This expectation derives from several sources. One source is the existence of pensions and Social Security benefits, which provide a replacement for wages. Earlier studies reported a custom among nonpension firms to retain older workers in nondemanding jobs to provide an income for them. Since the elderly now have other sources of income, they have less need of job income than they did in previous eras. Moreover, since they have access to such programs that the young do not have, the elderly need job income less than do the young. There may also be an expectation that the elderly should live at a lower standard of living than others.

Furthermore, there is a cultural expectation that the elderly need not support younger members of their families, and so have diminished need for income. For example, if an employer retires a grandfather so that a father can keep working, on the belief that the latter has greater need for the job to support his young children, the belief rests on the assumption made in our culture that fathers but not grandfathers have a duty to work to support the young ones of the family.

Retirement can also be seen simply as one instance of age stratification, the assignment of varying social roles to different age cohorts. The practice is common in some primitive societies; we use it for education, assigning student roles to youth.[23]

Finally, retirement can be seen as part of a specific belief in the fairness of an age-stratified pattern of career course in large, stable companies. In that pattern, one is hired into the firm while young, progresses up a ladder of promotions, and is retired when older so as to make room to promote others.

Apart from beliefs that such a system is economically efficient, it may be thought of as just. There is research consistent with this theory, reporting the attitudes of older workers and of personnel managers.[24] Nevertheless, an overwhelming majority of Americans do not believe mandatory retirement to be just.[25]

Cultural Devaluing and Ageism

Cultural reasons may exist for disrespect or ambivalence toward the elderly.[26] Under conditions of modernization, new jobs are created, often requiring new skills which are usually held by the young; with migration to the city there is a breakdown of the ties of the extended family; superior education is extended to the young; and there is, perhaps for these reasons, a cult of youth.[27] In addition, in a country like the United States, the chain of family tradition has been broken: each family is descended from immigrants who themselves left parental authority to come parentless to start a family line.[28] These cultural trends, like psychological causes, suggest that negative stereotypes of the aged may come to exist alongside the traditional positive images of the elderly. These beliefs may influence personnel decisions on the elderly. In this model, the situation of the aged may approximate that of women, who are also objects of ambivalence—with cultural and psychological sources— and are victims of stereotyping.

There is little support for the hypothesis that there is overt hostility toward the elderly. There has not been research suitable to test the causal hypothesis of unconscious ambivalence, nor to detect possible sources of variation in its strength over the decades due to shifting family constellations. Speculation as to the unconscious meaning of our treatment of the elderly still must rest upon clues and hints supplied by cultural data and by intuition.

Work-place Psychology

Individualized determination of worker competence may not be objectively difficult, but it may be subjectively difficult, and it may be difficult to justify to workers and their representatives. Unions apparently sometimes fight harder on individual grievances for specific older workers than they do against proposals to institute generalized mandatory retirement. Individual grievances may be fought hard because they involve a worker of high seniority adamant that he is still able. Generalized policies may be relatively more acceptable for several reasons: they obviate the need for individualized monitoring of performance, satisfying the wishes of many workers, and they are set at ages acceptable to most older workers. (The policies may also be acceptable because they are usually part of a pension package providing compensating benefits to older workers; by retiring high-seniority workers they open up jobs for younger workers; and in any case, such policies can be traded off as part of overall bargaining.) Moreover, even if unions do not fight grievances harder than general policies, since there are more grievances, management may find it less costly in terms of management time and trouble to handle the subject through bargaining about general policies.

Similar considerations apply also to some nonunion situations. Civil service hearings may be as burdensome to a government manager as union grievances are for a private manager, and so government employers without unions may prefer the general policy because they expect heavier costs in justifying individualized determinations than in promulgating a general policy.

All these explanations may point to an overall tendency toward routinization of decisions in large bureaucracies. In large firms, central management cannot easily supervise a system of individualized determination of retirement. Union leadership and management may both prefer uniform, firm-wide policies. Those who design pension plans may also find calculations simpler if there is a uniform retirement date. Uniform policies, such as discharge at a fixed age instead of when unfitness is determined individually, trade off different kinds of arbitrariness, fairness, and moral costs.

Conclusions

In the light of the studies that I have reviewed, some conclusions may now be set out on the causes of age-work policies such as mandatory retirement.

The substantively rational explanation, that employers retire the elderly because their productivity generally diminishes significantly at about the age of usual retirement, seems to have influenced many employers to have adopted such policies. To a large extent such a belief is inaccurate, but our inquiry then regresses one step to seek explanations for the belief. The posit of economic rationality does not explain why firms should act on an unsupported belief to discharge able workers.

In fact, it seems there was no research factually validating the belief in older workers' low productivity at the time mandatory retirement was instituted. Moreover, changes in retirement policies were made without benefit of changed data. Mandatory retirement policies were promulgated in a period when the elderly were thought to be "used up," but apparently that idea was not supported by any empirical studies. (Of course, the vast majority of business decisions—when to buy, when to sell, how much to pay, etc.—are made without benefit of systematic social science research, and there seems to be no special reason for hiring policies to be any different.)

The policies were continued by some employers who ignored the experience of other employers to the contrary, while the latter were retaining older workers and finding them generally able. When Social Security benefits became available, many employers made significant shifts in the retirement age—particularly as to women—without any new information on productivity. And when Congress voted to prohibit mandatory retirement at age 65, and then at any age, new empirical research on the work capacity of older workers was only one of many factors.

A second substantive rationality theory emphasizes not that older workers' productivity decreases, but that their wages increase. If workers receive a regular age bonus, it seems logical that at some age they will be paid more than their current production is worth. Yet the figures comparing firms with age-work policies and those without them do not seem to reveal differentially higher pay of older workers subject to retirement.

A separate substantive rationality explanation applies to bars against hiring of older persons. At one time such hiring could lead to disproportionate pension costs to firms, but this is no longer so under typical current pension arrangements. Some employers also feared that older workers had disproportionate accident rates, again without adequate empirical support and contrary to the experience of other firms.

Decisions on retirement policies thus do not seem to have been driven by profit-maximizing employer behavior responding to diminished worker productivity or productivity/wage ratio.

Explanations in terms of process rationality fall with the substantive ones. If there is no general failure around age 65 of workers' abilities to do their jobs, then the need for measurement at that age is not acute. Moreover, there are data suggesting that employers are indeed able to identify individual submarginal workers both before and after the usual retirement age. In almost nine out of ten firms with mandatory retirement, as in both the major Supreme Court mandatory retirement cases, the employer had in place systems to determine worker capacity or achievement.[29] As the trial judge found in *Murgia,* it simply is not rational to let go a worker of demonstrated individual capacity because of a generalization about workers' usual low competence.[30] More significant may be another version of a process rationality explanation—the psychology of the process.

The systemic rationality argument, though a common one and widely believed by the current cohort of personnel managers, seems a makeweight. A mandatory retirement system may enhance morale among younger workers who get quicker promotions, but it may reduce the morale of older workers facing imminent retirement. Moreover, an ambitious younger worker can be rewarded even if an older worker continues to occupy some job slot: he or she can be given salary increases, better titles, or increased responsibilities. Furthermore, if industry in general abolishes compulsory retirement (as happens when the decision is made by legislation), then ambitious younger workers are less likely to switch firms over this issue, thus decreasing its significance to management. Additionally, a systemic preference for job rotation would seem to call for a limit on tenure in a given job, rather than an age-based rule retiring the worker from the firm. Turnover, not retirement, seems the key concern. Voluntary retirement has a much larger quantitative effect on the work force than does mandatory retirement and can be encouraged by appropriate pension benefits and by planning measures that encourage an expectation of a usual time of retirement while permitting individuals to opt for longer work.

Finally, the quantitative significance of the systemic value of forced retirement seems small. Studies have shown that only a small fraction of the work force reaching age 65 wants to continue work, is able to work, and was forced out by nonindividualized compulsory retirement. Furthermore, if such persons continue working, on the average the number of years of continued employment for each person is small. Thus, the incremental average delay in opening up positions in general that flows from a policy change is minor. The number involved is so small (a fraction of 1% of the work force) that the quantitative effect is still low even when one includes a ripple effect of jobs opened up by promotions to fill retirement vacancies. Alternative personnel practices could more efficiently create openings through required transfers or rotation.

There is some evidence supporting the explanation of intergroup competition. Employer decisions on retirement policies are made in the context of the overall labor market. Older workers are let go only when there are younger workers available to fill the jobs; in labor shortages older workers are kept on longer than usual. Unions sometimes seek or acquiesce in mandatory retirement, particularly when unemployment is high. But younger workers have not generally been active in suggesting mandatory retirement policies, through unions or otherwise, except when great labor surpluses have existed.

An explanation as to why older workers, not others, are forced out of jobs in times of labor surplus involves a combination of factors, many of which involve the rationality factors already discussed. Because of the age bonus, older workers are generally paid more than younger ones. Because of cohort effects, younger workers may be better educated; the recent formal education of the young may be valued more than the accumulated experience of the old. Downward adjustment of the wages of the elderly may be difficult because of morale factors and union or civil service policies. There is in addition a widespread cultural idea that the elderly have less of a moral duty to work and less of a moral claim on their jobs because they have pensions available and because of the other reasons discussed above.

The explanation in terms of intertemporal choice has limited support. Survey data do show agreement with the idea that the aged should retire to make room for the young. It should be remembered, though, that when jobs are scarce, the joint effect of the seniority and retirement system protects the jobs of workers in their fifties and early sixties, while letting go older workers at a time when most workers would retire voluntarily. The net effect of these policies is thus to help, not harm, most older persons who are willing and able to work. At the same time there is currently widespread opposition, among both older and younger persons, to compulsory retirement and other practices that are seen as age discrimination.

Union policies have been significant in several of the points made thus far: the combination of union policies might be thought to drive management toward a policy of retirement at a uniform age. Unions have advocated seniority and age bonus systems, which raise the costs of employing older workers, and have also resisted lowering the wages of older workers as their productivity diminishes. They have also required management to go to lengths to justify individualized decisions on discharge for lessened productivity.

It should be noted, though, that unions have sometimes permitted older workers to be switched to other jobs at lower wages when they could no longer perform the jobs which they previously performed. Furthermore, it has not been the presence of unions per se that led to this combination of policies. Civil service systems in government departments without unionization also provide job protection to long-time employees, wage increases with longevity, protection against lowered wages, and procedural rights against individualized dismissal. The union policies are in part aggregations of individual preferences: grievances are hard-fought because individualized determinations are painful. Similarly, management avoidance of grievance procedures reflects in part the employer's own emotional discomfort at individualized determination of incapacity.

The range of retirement practices a society can afford is determined by overall labor supply and demand, productivity, and the dependency ratio. At the same time, a particular retirement policy can exist only when it is culturally acceptable. Mandatory retirement could not have been so easily instituted if there was militant opposition by older workers who perceived it as unfair. When there was serious political demand for its abolition by law, management resistance was not strong. Cultural attitudes as to whether and when workers should retire seem to have been important in determining what age-work policies were adopted within the range of the economically possible.

Age-based policies on appointment, promotion, or retirement often as-sume a certain "normal" career path. Age limits on entry-level jobs, for ex-ample, calculate from birth and not from entry into the job market, and thus do not make provision for women who seek work after childbearing and child-rearing. (On that reasoning, the English courts have held that company rules excluding job applicants above a certain age constitute indirect sex discrimi-nation.[31]) Pension eligibility is also calculated in years since birth and not in years left until the statistically predicted likely date of death. Thus, it does not provide for handicapped or minority persons who, though healthy, have a shorter life expectancy.

This discussion leads to an overall conclusion. The data do not establish that the existence and characteristics of age-work policies can be explained by the posit of rational profit-maximization by employers and workers. Mac-roeconomic factors do seem to have created a zone of feasible age-work prac-tices. The selection of policies within that range seems to have been driven in large measure by cultural and psychological factors—intergenerational atti-tudes and attitudes toward personnel decisions—rather than by a simple eco-nomic rationality. Managers who thought that older workers were inefficient were reflecting widespread, but unsupported, belief. Managers who thought that mandatory retirement was needed as part of a normal promotional process may have been largely influenced by cultural ideas of a "normal" career. De-cisions to adopt age-work policies may have brought no correction by the competitive market as long as the exclusion of older workers had an economic effect on the firm roughly equivalent to the exclusion of some other group of workers in time of labor surplus. Preferences associated with large firms, unions, or civil service may also have pushed firms away from individualized determinations toward a routinized system—involving uniform, bureaucratic policies of age bonuses and seniority rules, followed by cessation of seniority rights and mandatory retirement at a uniform date.

20 • Empirical Bases of Normative Judgment

From Description to Justification

We must understand mandatory retirement in order to judge it. The previous chapters, largely causal in focus, foreshadowed many normative concerns. Four types of explanatory models and their variants have been considered in this study as candidate causal factors to help in deciding just what kind of phenomenon mandatory retirement is. In seeking to describe and understand age-work social practices, I have surveyed empirical research and hypotheses and compared them with the set of models. When we turn from the empirical level to the normative, we consider the arguments based on these causal accounts that seek to justify the existence of age-related work policies. In going from description to justification, we may analyze the arguments in three steps.

First, a satisfactory normative account of age-work practices must be based on a valid empirical account of those practices. Thus, in order for any of the possible causes of age-work policies to serve as the basis for a satisfying justification, it must in fact be the operative cause for the adoption or retention of such policies. Considering the model of intergroup competition, for example, someone might argue that it would be justifiable to require retirement of the old so as to provide jobs for black workers. Such a justification is historically inapposite because that model does not fit the data on the causes for the adoption of age-work practices. And that justification remains irrelevant because it does not fit current data relating age-work practices to job openings.

Second, for a justification to work, the facts it assumes must also be accurate. When it is only a matter of causal explanations (our first step), belief may suffice: for example, if employers believed that older workers were less cost-effective, the belief would suffice to lead them to adopt age-work policies. But for the causally operative explanation to be normatively satisfactory as a justification, it must (as a second step) rest on true rather than false factual beliefs. The relevant causal belief can be a satisfactory justification only if the factual premises on which it is based are accurate. For example, retiring the old if they are no longer competent might be normatively justified, but the justification fails if in fact they are competent. The evidence reviewed in Part 3 shows little reason to accept the belief that most persons around typical retirement age who wish to continue work fall below acceptable performance levels at their jobs. Thus, the substantive rationality model, since it involves unsupported negative beliefs (stereotypes) does not provide a general justification for mandatory retirement, even if it supplies an explanation. The process rationality model falls with the substantive rationality ones.

As a third step in normative judgment, a particular empirical explanation of age-work practices, even if causally operative and factually based, still must be of the kind that provides a normative justification of the practice. Our standards of permissible normative justifications may, depending on the context of judgment, be drawn from general morality, from constitutional law, or from statutes. Thus, if an attitudinal model of hostility to the aged explains the adoption of age-work policies, that explanation could be rejected as the basis for a justification.

Other empirical data are also relevant to the normative analysis because they specify the harm caused by the practice in question. The replacement ratio of pension income to prior wages indicates whether workers suffer severe economic loss at retirement. The fraction of employers with age-work policies determines whether workers in a given industry have a realistic choice between firms with and without mandatory retirement.

The Research Agenda

The findings of social science research can help inform legal decision, and legal doctrine in turn can help define issues for social science research. Age-work policy is made by legal-decision makers—legislatures, courts, and administrative agencies—as well as by businesses and unions. All have an important need for empirical information on the topics reviewed in this work. That need should help shape the research agenda.

Federal Policy Research

Congressional action on age-work policies has been driven, we may assume, by political realities and by a sense of the public good, rather than by increases in scientific knowledge.[1] Nevertheless, at several key points in the process Congress, perhaps to delay difficult political decisions, has mandated the administration to study the empirical base of its age-work policy choices. Thus, section 715 of the Civil Rights Act of 1964 directed the Secretary of Labor to "make a full and complete study of the factors which might tend to result in discrimination in employment because of age and of the consequences of such discrimination on the economy and individuals affected."[2] The resulting report, *The Older American Worker,* identified "arbitrary dis-

167

crimination" that rejected older workers because of assumptions about the effect of age on ability, when there is in fact no basis for those assumptions.[3]

The 1967 ADEA Amendments, in section 5, directed the Secretary of Labor "to undertake an appropriate study of institutional and other arrangements giving rise to involuntary retirement."[4] A resulting report, the 1973 Employer Practices Survey by the Bureau of Labor Statistics, showed that about half of the private nonagricultural labor force was subject to mandatory retirement practices.[5]

The 1978 ADEA Amendments required the Labor Department to examine the consequences, for both workers and firms, of raising the mandatory retirement age to 70; to evaluate the feasibility of raising or eliminating this age; and to study the effects of the executive and tenured faculty exceptions in the act. The federal government's Office of Personnel Management was also directed to study the effects of uncapping the ADEA's protection for most federal employees.[6] The Labor Department report submitted to Congress was *The Age Discrimination in Employment Act Studies* that have been discussed extensively.

The 1986 ADEA Amendments called for further studies dealing with two time-limited exceptions to the abolition of mandatory retirement.[7] In the language we have been using, the studies would deal with the systemic rationality justifications for a tenured faculty exception, and the process rationality justification for a police and firefighter exception.

Future Research

The conclusions put forward in this work may lead to future research, using the typology of causes of age-work practices and the list of their characteristics as frameworks for additional empirical and historical studies or for meta-analysis of previous work. The studies to date cannot support conclusively any of the explanations for age-work policies in the typology, nor do they fully solve the puzzle of the characteristics of age-work practices.

More research is needed on workers over age 70. For example, for workers over age 70 who are employed and wish to continue to work, when are there common significant drops in productivity? How is the answer different for different occupations, different working conditions, different cohorts? How does their productivity/earnings ratio compare with that of younger workers? Could changed assignments, work conditions, self-pacing, and the like be cost-effective in enhancing their productivity? How many workers (and which unions) would be open to a revised compensation basis for older workers that restored an acceptable productivity/earnings ratio? Are existing systems for individualized determination of health or productivity for different types of workers acceptable in terms of accuracy and cost? How can the psychic costs of such determinations best be minimized? Which flexible systems for individualized partial or phased retirement are most welcome to both employees and firms? What alternatives to mandatory retirement have proven workable in various types of firms to serve the purpose of keeping open the channels of promotion?

Limitations on the Policy Use of Research

Research of this type will not solve all age-work problems for our society. American legal scholars half a century ago embraced social science with the hope that it had answers to the questions law asked, so that an objective basis could be found on which to build social policy. Nowadays the law has more limited hopes.[8]

Much of social and biological science, in gerontology as in other areas, deals with matters not directly relevant to legal issues. When studies are relevant, they may still be laboratory experiments lacking the ecological validity that would justify expanding their conclusions to real-world situations. Even if the studies apply directly to real-life situations, there will still be few definitive answers.

And even the clearest answers may not be "objective" in any simple sense of that term. Knowledge is acquired in a social context: choice of topic and level of inquiry, framing of issues and selection of methodology, interpretation of results—all provide ample room for personal and social preferences, blind spots, and fears and wishes (both conscious and unconscious) to influence the reported results.

Even ideal research, moreover, can hardly be expected to shape public-policy choices in any direct way. Public-policy decisions—in courts as well as in legislatures—is still based upon interests, aspirations, and tradition as well as upon knowledge. And the decisions are formed through compromise and incrementalism more than they are wrought in any straightforward selection of means toward clear ends.

Additionally, applied research is used in political and adversarial contexts. While legislative bodies and courts sometimes have institutional ways of commissioning or receiving social science research, even such bodies may not be what social scientists regard as "objective." Furthermore, American legislatures and common-law courts traditionally rely on admitted partisans—interest groups, litigants, or individual legislators—to develop or communicate pertinent information. In such applied contexts, research questions may be framed in terms of the support available for specific legally significant propositions, rather than in terms of testing neutral hypotheses or building models. Researchers may find that their potential audience (which will first have to be educated as to the existence of relevant scholars and methods) may define questions that are both more specific and more slanted than is usual in the academic world and may require answers on timetables far more rapid than academic research usually observes.

Furthermore, even ideal research provided to ideal decision-makers may only frame choices rather than dictating them, leaving an irreducible core of the necessity for value choice. Whether these value choices are made by the framers of the Constitution, by the legislature, by the executive branch, or by the courts, value choices remain to be made even after the facts are known.

After all is said, understanding of the facts is an important part of the formulation of public policy, and research, with all its limitations, has an important role in checking the pictures of the world otherwise supplied by common sense. The existing knowledge reviewed in this book, for example, while not answering all age-work policy questions, does undercut many of the common justifications given for accepted practice. Knowledge thus serves at the least to sharpen policy choices, guiding though not dictating choice, and limiting the range of options. Further research on age-work questions will be important in helping decide the policy questions on tomorrow's agenda.

Epilogue

Like other ongoing social inequalities, age-work practices have been defended through justifications that attract wide support. The conclusion of this work is that, as general justifications, both the common-sense and the scholarly defenses of age-based mandatory retirement fall short.

The practice may nevertheless be justified for some jobs in some industries during some periods. The U.S. Courts, accepting the premises of the Age Discrimination in Employment Act, allow an age-based retirement rule if all workers of that age are unsuitable for the position, or if most are and it is impractical to test individually. And the same Congress that adopted in 1986 a general prohibition of age-based mandatory retirement nevertheless retained some exceptions to that prohibition, pending further study.

The bases for the specific 1986 statutory exceptions are instructive. An exception is allowed when personnel decision-making is properly allocated to some process other than general legislation (i.e., as regards the internal employees of Congress itself). Another is allowed when it is highly likely that older workers will be unsuitable, when the risks to public safety are great, and when the expense of case-by-case justification of policies is high (i.e., with local police and firefighters). Still another special case occurs when, because of period effects and the special circumstances of one line of work, there is a perceived need to keep up retirements to provide openings for new hires (i.e., with tenured university professors). What must be emphasized is that all these instances where mandatory retirement was excluded from legal prohibition were regarded by Congress as temporary, based on special circumstances, and subject to actual proof. Broad-brush justifications of age-work policies, which this study concludes to be unwarranted, have been rejected by a virtually unanimous Congress.

Retirement and the Sabbath

Turning from these conclusions, it is interesting to consider retirement policies against a wider tapestry. Some think that retirement was made possible only by the extension of average lifespan in modern times. Enhanced longevity is, in turn, largely a product of better nutrition, improved public health, and substantial elimination of the traditional epidemics and of death in child-birth.[1] In earlier times, most people worked as long as they lived. It is only in modern times that parents can complete the tasks of childrearing—and that most women survive childbearing—and still have years of healthy life ahead of them.[2] Some believe that in modern times retirement is limited, on the other hand, by the changing dependency ratio; as the proportion of workers and re-tired persons changes, there is a graying of the population. Because of the increase in the fraction of the population that is elderly, there is now a move-ment to limit retirement and to delay eligibility for Social Security. These views suggest that retirement as a social phenomenon could thrive only within a relatively narrow window, the time span between two phenomena each unique in the history of the world: the lengthening of life and the graying of the population.

Longer life span is not, however, a necessary prerequisite of a retirement system; a short-lived people could have the practice of retirement. Nor is the dependency ratio a necessary limit to it: a society could decide to support a large fraction of nonworking elders. It is a normative decision within a culture as to how much consumption will be allocated to the elderly. The decision will be influenced by the gross national product of the society. Total social produc-tion is influenced not only by the life span, retirement age, or dependency ratio, but depends also on productivity and endowment of natural resources. There are also many alternate social provisions for adjusting the number of worker-hours in society—length of work day and work week, length of an-nual vacations, starting age for work, and the custom as to work by women.

The institution of retirement, in principle, is made possible by improved productivity, capture of labor surplus by workers, and trade-offs between con-sumption and leisure, which in combination enable society to support a sub-stantial fraction of nonworkers. The institution of retirement then represents intertemporal life-cycle choices allocating that leisure to the later stages of life. Industrialization and its improved productivity have made it possible for society to support a given level of consumption with fewer worker-hours of effort. Workers in the industrialized West have won the allocation to them of a substantial portion of the value of their production. Much of that value is chosen to be taken as leisure.

How that leisure is typically allocated within the life cycle varies among cultures. The leisure possible to workers can be taken through less than full exertion each hour of work, historically the oldest method known to laborers. It can also be taken as fewer hours worked each day or fewer days worked each week—the historical Sabbath. Fewer weeks can be worked per year, providing vacations for the laboring force. Or fewer years can be worked in a lifetime, with one's life work starting later or retirement occurring earlier. Retirement can thus be seen as just a different form of allocation of the available leisure time, forming a series with the Sabbath rest invented three millennia ago and with the workday reforms of the nineteenth and twentieth centuries. Retirement is another form of Sabbath.

The term *Sabbath* (in Hebrew, *shabbat*) probably was originally a common noun for a time of rest. The term is used in the Bible not just for the seventh day but also for several holidays and even for the sabbatical year.[3] The adoption by the Hebrews of a weekly day of rest was controversial in antiquity; though other ancient peoples had rest days (the Egyptians are said to have rested twice a month, at new moon and full moon), no one else had weekly rests.[4] We can see the seventh-day rest as an early step in the long series of attempts to provide workers with *shabbaton*, times of rest.

Seeing retirement as a form of Sabbath gives another meaning to its being obligatory. Many other rests for workers, from the original Sabbath through some of the modern restrictions, have been phrased in mandatory terms. The age-old tradition of prescriptions of rest from work may have been an additional component lending acceptance to the mandatory characteristic of the modern institution of retirement.

In the modern era there has been a growth in leisure by a reduction of the labor force at both ends of the working life. The movement to delay the start of work by adolescents, for example, enjoyed major support from unions and was institutionalized in child-labor laws and compulsory school attendance. The increase in nonworking years has been about nine years in the United States in this century. That amount, though, is only about one-third the amount of free time added through work-week reductions and longer vacations.[5] Like the child-labor changes, these reductions were also won largely by unions. Restrictions on hours worked per day and per week were also institutionalized through laws, primarily those requiring time-and-a-half pay for overtime work. In Europe, as contrasted to the United States, there is an even greater tendency to lengthen the weekend and vacation rather than to increase nonworking years by retiring earlier and starting work later.[6]

The increase in nonworking years in thus less significant than other increases in time off. Furthermore, it has been more than offset by an increase in *working* years within the longer usual life span. Though U.S. workers in the 1960s worked 1,200 hours *per year* less than those of the 1890s, they still worked a total of 6,800 hours more *in their lifetime*.[7]

Pension schemes serve to smooth lifetime earnings roughly in accordance with family needs throughout the life cycle. A somewhat more even distribution of income throughout the life span may increase the total utility of lifetime earnings. This smoothing is often achieved through voluntary savings, but persons with high time-preference for goods will save little while earning. A pension plan may function for them as a paternalistic policy imposing forced savings, increasing utility during postwork years and thus maximizing total lifetime satisfaction.

Under conditions of involuntary retirement, however, the individual is unable to convert free time into income even when that would maximize her satisfactions. Free time has little utility when it is perceived as excessive; an uneven distribution over the states of life of leisure and work (with its associated income and the availability of goods) will then fail to maximize satisfactions.[8]

The allocation of leisure is simultaneously an allocation of work. If one believes that there is only so much work to go around (a limited labor fund or "lump of labor"), then the Sabbath, retirement, and other reductions in hours that each employee works are valued as providing opportunity for other laborers to have jobs. If one thinks that a system of promotions will go smoothly only if older workers can be forced from their jobs, then mandatory retirement is valued as providing promotional opportunities. If those economic theories are rejected, however, then retirement, like the Sabbath, is valued as providing a break from the demands of work. Whatever the merits of a compulsory Sabbath, compulsory retirement is then seen as unjustified.

Education and Compulsion

The conclusion we have reached as to the causes of age-work practices does not fully support Congress's assumption that the age-work effect should be analogized with racial differentiation in employment and treated as "discrimination." As Congress realized when passing the 1978 ADEA Amendments,[9] stereotype rather than overt hostility is the problem. For all that we know so far about age-work practices, some might argue that it would have been a generally sufficient remedy if the government documented for employers the capacities of older workers and the experience of firms without mandatory retirement. A public relations program supplying that information widely to employers might have convinced them that their economic best interests dictated abandonment of across-the-board retirement rules. From this point of view, the key parts of the ADEA are sections 2 and 3, adopting findings of fact and establishing an education program, and some might question why there was any need for section 7, the enforcement provision.

An educational approach was recommended in the Secretary of Labor's 1965 report[10] and has been tried in other countries. Several governments were particularly concerned to overcome employer prejudice based on age by promoting studies "to show that, in most cases, such prejudices result from inconclusive or erroneous information."[11] The Canadian government, for example, has been quite active, more or less continuously since the end of World War II, in educational publicity to combat age discrimination against older workers. It has given wide publicity to government pamphlets, articles, and broadcasts; news stories; and a film called *Date of Birth*. Several European countries also actively encourage the employment of older workers. Some success was reported by both Great Britain and Canada for their official educational and publicity campaigns in achieving declining prejudice among employers against hiring older workers. Results of efforts in other countries are largely unavailable.

It is highly significant, from this viewpoint, that the ADEA also includes section 7(d): "The Secretary . . . shall promptly seek to eliminate any alleged unlawful practice by informal methods of conciliation, conference, and persuasion."[12] The employer who refuses settlement—who insists on mandatory retirement even though age is not a bona fide occupational qualification[13]—presumably is not accepting a rational employment policy. There is then (if not before) reason to suspect that bias is at work. The age discrimination concept embodied in the statute is an apt one for dealing with employers who resist persuasion. The law's compulsory enforcement measures to fight such age discrimination thus are justifiable.

The empirical conclusion reached here does not support the Supreme Court's assumption that the age-work effect exists for reasons of substantive and process economic rationality.[14] The very cases before the Supreme Court involved employers who (like nine out of ten retirement firms) had systems in place for individualized determination of capacity or performance and dealt with older workers who had been individually determined to be still capable.[15] The Court conceded, for example, that there was "no dispute" that Murgia was "capable of performing the duties of a uniformed officer." The Court's belief that mandatory retirement under such conditions is economically rational remains merely an assumption. Indeed, its statements about the elderly seem to reflect the same stereotypes upon which it was called to pass judgment.[16]

The research reviewed in this study is thus of value to the ongoing policy debate on whether mandatory retirement should properly be treated as age discrimination, a question on which Congress and the Supreme Court have reached conflicting answers.[17] The typology of causes of age-work policies has been useful in comparing various age-work theories, and the list of characteristics of age-work policies has been useful in checking whether those theories satisfactorily account for the policies.

The Golden Bough and the Golden Years

As we reach the end of this work, we can spend a moment speculating on the psychological and cultural factors that seem to have been such important contributing causes to age-work practices. We do not have hard data enabling us to know with certainty the underlying meaning of these practices, but we observe that employers used them to force many of the elderly from their work roles, thinking that dead wood must be cut away to make room for the strong next generation, while using age-work practices to avoid the pain of individualized removal.

Have people's feelings about such practices left traces in the anthropological and mythical records of common human emotions? If we go to the bookshelf, we can reread a famous passage:

> Down to the decline of Rome a custom was observed at Nemi which seems to transport us at once from civilization to savagery. In the sacred grove there grew a certain tree round which at any time of the day, and probably far into the night, a grim figure might be seen to prowl. In his hand he carried a drawn sword, and he kept peering warily about him as if at every instant he expected to be set upon by an enemy. He was a priest and a murderer; and the man for whom he looked was sooner or later to murder him and hold the priesthood in his stead. Such was the rule of the sanctuary. A candidate for the priesthood could only succeed to office by slaying the priest, and having slain him, he retained office till he was himself slain by a stronger or a craftier. The post which he held by this precarious tenure carried with it the title of king.[18]

Thus Sir James G. Frazer began his famed anthropological work, *The Golden Bough.* He began with a line in Virgil; an explanation was suggested to him by "similar rules formerly imposed on kings in Southern India";[19] he went on to collect fourteen volumes of related customs and myths from all over the world. Frazer sought to demonstrate universal themes and motives inherent in that ancient tale of the sacred king.

Even without opening Frazer's work, those who remember their classical mythology will recall the strange tale that the ruler god Uranus was conquered, castrated, and succeeded by his son Cronus (Saturn). Cronus was in turn dethroned and hurled from the top of Olympus by his son Zeus (Jupiter), who replaced him as chief of the gods. And Zeus was warned by prophecy to be on guard against being overthrown by his own child, and so took cannibalistic precautionary steps. So too the ancient Greek tale of Oedipus, with its version of the son who kills his father to succeed to the kingship, captured the attention of many long before Freud. And in his speculations in *Totem and Taboo,* Freud wondered whether murder of the father to succeed to his privileges might not have been an archaic pattern.[20]

The social function of myths, set in the form of stories of a legendary past, is to give meaning to ordinary social institutions. There is a long tradition, of which Frazer and Freud were part, of using this particular set of old stories as part of new arguments. Perhaps I can be forgiven for finding in them legendary depictions of an institution of retirement. If not in social reality, at least in cultural ideas, many peoples at varied times and places have had the thought that patriarchal rulers may be displaced by their successors of the next generation through murder.

It was not until our own era that is was common for the older generation to live long enough, in large enough numbers, that retirement became a general issue. The anthropological and classical myths are hints supporting the idea that people might feel that forced retirement of the elderly was something like murder. Like the ancients, we often may have felt that to achieve our own success we would have to force out the fathers—if not kill, at least shove to the wayside. An action with such meaning might well generate anxiety.

The age-work practice of using an impersonal rule to force retirements serves to avoid personal responsibility, so binding and limiting that anxiety. To avoid facing the harms and injustices of forced retirement, we have also had our own quasi-myths—the Gold Watch that supposedly honored and rewarded the retired worker, and the Golden Years of retirement in which he would enjoy leisure and happiness. America today, in rejecting forced retirement, seeks a world in which at last Frazer's *Golden Bough* is abandoned, and elders no longer need be forcibly cast aside to make room for the succeeding generation.

Notes

Chapter 1.   Equality and Age-Work Practices

1. N.Y. Educ. Law, § 239 (Consol. 1985).
2. Weiss v. Walsh, 324 F. Supp. 75 (S.D.N.Y. 1971), *aff'd*, 461 F.2d 846 (2d Cir. 1972), *cert. denied*, 409 U.S. 1129 (1973), *reh'g. denied*, 410 U.S. 970 (1973).
3. Massachusetts Bd. of Retirement v. Murgia, 427 U.S. 307 (1976).
4. Vance v. Bradley, 440 U.S. 93, 107–10 (1979).
5. *Working Americans: Equality at Any Age,* Hearings before the Senate Special Committee on Aging, 99th Cong., 2d sess., 1986, 143 (statement of Burton Fretz, executive director, National Senior Citizens Law Center).
6. International Labor Office, *Report of the Director General,* pt. 1 (1962).
7. Dorothy P. Rice, "Foreword" in *Aging,* ed. Aliza Kolker and Paul Ahmed (New York: Elsevier Science Publishing Co., 1982), xi; National Council on Aging, *Fact Book on Aging: A Profile of America's Older Population* (Washington, D.C.: National Council on Aging, 1978), 104; Clark Tibbitts, "Preface," in *Handbook of Social Gerontology,* ed. Clark Tibbitts (Chicago: University of Chicago Press, 1960); Martin L. Levine, "The Emergence of Special Rights for the Elderly in National Law around the World," in *More to Life: Proceedings of the XI International Conference of Gerontology* (Paris: International Center for Social Gerontology, forthcoming).
8. Martin L. Levine, "The Frame of Nature, Gerontology, and the Law," *Southern California Law Review* 56 (1982): 26.
9. Age Discrimination in Employment Act of 1967, Pub. L. No. 90-202, 81 Stat. 602 (codified as amended 29 U.S.C.A. §§ 621–34 (West Supp. 1987)). Also the Age Discrimination Act of 1975, Pub. L. No. 94–135, 89 Stat. 728–32 (codified as amended at 42 U.S.C.A. §§ 6101–7 (West Supp. 1987)); Comprehensive Older Americans Act Amendments of 1978, Pub. L. No. 95–478, 92 Stat. 1513 (codified as amended in scattered sections of 42 U.S.C.A. (West Supp. 1987)).
10. G. Boglietti, "Discrimination against Older Workers and the Promotion of Equality and Opportunity," *International Labour Review* 110 (1974): 351–52.
11. Peter Schuck, "The Graying of Civil Rights Law: The Age Discrimination Act of 1975," *Yale Law Journal* 89 (1979): 27; Lawrence M. Friedman, *Your Time Will Come: The Law of Age Discrimination and Mandatory Retirement* (New York: Russell Sage Foundation, 1984).
12. Massachusetts Bd. of Retirement v. Murgia, 427 U.S. 307 (1976); Vance v. Bradley, 440 U.S. 93 (1979).

13. Martin Levine, "Four Models for Age/Work Policy Research," *Gerontologist* 20 (October 1980): 561–74.
14. Charles Lund Black, *Structure and Relationship in Constitutional Law* (Baton Rouge: Louisiana State University Press, 1969).
15. Massachusetts Bd. of Retirement v. Murgia, 427 U.S. 307, 313 (1976).
16. Age Discrimination in Employment Act Amendments of 1978, Pub. L. No. 95–256, 92 Stat. 189 (codified as amended at 29 U.S.C.A. §§ 623–34 (West Supp. 1987)).
17. Age Discrimination in Employment Act Amendments of 1986, Pub. L. No. 99–592, 100 Stat. 3342, 29 U.S.C.A. §§ 622–24, 630–31 (West Supp. 1987).
18. Select Committee on Aging, *Eliminating Mandatory Retirement*, 99th Cong., 2d sess., 1986, Committee Print, 4.
19. Comment, "Age Discrimination in Employment Act Amendments of 1978: Tension between Congress and the Courts," *Brigham Young University Law Review*, 1980, 570–71.
20. Massachusetts Bd. of Retirement v. Murgia, 427 U.S. 307, 312–13.
21. See Martin L. Levine, "Comments on the Constitutional Law of Age Discrimination," *Chicago-Kent Law Review* 55 (1979): 1081.
22. Cf. United Air Lines v. McMann, 434 U.S. 192 (1977) with Western Air Lines, Inc. v. Criswell, 472 U.S. 400 (1985), and Johnson v. Mayor and City Council of Baltimore, 472 U.S. 353 (1985).
23. Richard A. Posner, *The Economics of Justice* (Cambridge: Harvard University Press, 1981), 368, n. 12.
24. Lester C. Thurow, *Generating Inequality: Mechanisms of Distribution in the U.S. Economy* (New York: Basic Books, 1975), sec. 9.
25. Gary S. Becker, *The Economics of Discrimination*, 2d ed. (Chicago: University of Chicago Press, 1971).
26. Peter Schuck, "Age Discrimination Revisited," *Chicago-Kent Law Review* 57 (1981): 1035–36.
27. Note by Amy Wax, "Waiver of Rights under the Age Discrimination in Employment Act of 1967," *Columbia Law Review* 86 (1986): 1086, n. 116.
28. Note, "The Age Discrimination in Employment Act of 1967," *Harvard Law Review* 90 (1976): 395–98.
29. Such claims include Frontiero v. Richardson, 411 U.S. 677 (1973) (plurality opinion); Craig v. Boren, 429 U.S. 190 (1976). On age discrimination see Martin L. Levine, "Age Discrimination as a Legal Concept for Analyzing Age-Work Issues," in *Work and Retirement: Policy Issues*, ed. Pauline K. Ragan (Los Angeles: University of Southern California Press, 1980), 45. See generally Charles D. Edelman and Ilene C. Siegler, *Federal Age Discrimination in Employment Law: Slowing Down the Gold Watch* (Charlottesville, Va.: Michie Co., 1978); Howard C. Eglit, *Age Discrimination*, 3 vols. (Colorado Springs: Shepard's/McGraw-Hill, 1986), vol. 2.

Age discrimination is a key issue in the new field of law and aging. See the following discussions by Martin L. Levine: "Legal Education and Curriculum Reform: 'Law and Aging' as a New Legal Field," *Minnesota Law Review* 65

(1981): 2671; "Research in Law and Aging," *Gerontologist* 20 (April 1980): 163–67; *Elderlaw: Legal, Ethical, and Policy Issues of Older Individuals and an Aging Society—Cases and Materials* (Washington, D.C.: Legal Services Corp., 1988); "Introduction: The Frame of Nature, Gerontology, and Law," *Southern California Law Review* 56 (1982): 261–88.

30. See, e.g., Frank J. Michelman, "On Protecting the Poor through the Fourteenth Amendment," *Harvard Law Review* 83 (1969): 7–59; the Supreme Court rejected the argument that statutes which discriminate against the poor should be subject to heightened scrutiny under the Fourteenth Amendment in Dandridge v. Williams, 397 U.S. 471 (1970). See also Note, "Mental Illness: A Suspect Classification?" *Yale Law Journal* 83 (1974): 1237–70, and Note, "The Equal Protection Clause and Exclusionary Zoning after Valtierra and Dandridge," *Yale Law Journal* 81 (1971): 61–86.

31. Matilda White Riley, Marilyn E. Johnson, and Anne Foner, *A Sociology of Age Stratification*, vol. 3 of *Aging and Society* (New York: Russell Sage Foundation, 1972), 402.

32. Eglit, *Age Discrimination*, 1: 1-1; also see Leonard D. Cain, "The Growing Importance of Legal Age in Determining the Status of the Elderly," *Gerontologist* 14 (1974): 167.

33. House Select Committee on Aging, *Age Stereotypes and Television*, 95th Cong., 1st sess., 1977, Committee Print; Neil S. Lutsky, "Attitudes toward Old Age and Elderly Persons," *Annual Review of Gerontology and Geriatrics* 1 (1980): 287.

34. Eglit, *Age Discrimination*, vol. 1, sec. 8.

35. City of Cleburne v. Cleburne Living Center, Inc., 473 U.S. 432, 455 (1985) (Marshall, J., with Brennan and Blackmun, JJ., dissenting).

36. E.g., 22 U.S.C. § 4052 (foreign service officers) and 14 C.F.R. §121.383(c) (airline pilots).

37. Robert Elmore, "The Older Worker and Age Discrimination," *Journal of Business Law*, 1980, 406.

38. William Safire, "The Codgerdoggle," *New York Times*, 3 Sept. 1977, 29, cited in Jeffrey Sonnenfeld, "Dealing with the Aging Work Force," *Harvard Business Review* 56 (November–December 1978): 85.

39. *Murgia*, 427 U.S. at 315.

40. *Vance*, 440 U.S. at 112.

41. Chief Justice Burger (born 1907), Justice Brennan (born 1906), Justice Marshall (born 1908), Justice Blackmun (born 1908), and Justice Powell (born 1907). Justice White, author of the majority opinion, was born in 1917. Gerald Gunther, *Cases and Materials on Constitutional Law* (Mineola, N.Y.: Foundation Press, 1980), A-7.

42. *Vance*, 440 U.S. at 107–10.

43. The District Court granted summary judgment for the plaintiffs. Bradley v. Vance, 436 F. Supp. 134 (D.D.C. 1977); *Vance*, 440 U.S. at 95.

44. State v. Noll, 444 U.S. 1007 (1980).

45. Oliver Wendell Holmes, "The Deacon's Masterpiece; or, The Wonderful One-

Hoss Shay," in *The Autocrat of the Breakfast-Table* (Boston: Houghton Mifflin, 1886), 252–53, 256.

46. James F. Fries and Lawrence M. Crapo, *Vitality and Aging: Implications of the Rectangular Curve* (San Francisco: Freeman, 1981).

47. Quoted in Lissy F. Jarvik, "Discussion: Patterns of Intellectual Functioning in the Later Years," in *Intellectual Functioning in Adults*, ed. Lissy F. Jarvik, Carl Eisdorfer, and June E. Blum (New York: Springer, 1973), 66.

48. 29 U.S.C.A. § 623(f)(1) (West Supp. 1987).

49. Usery v. Tamiami Trail Tours, Inc., 531 F. 2d 224, 235 (5th Cir. 1976); Western Air Lines, Inc., v. Criswell, 472 U.S. 400 (1985).

50. Bernice Neugarten, "Age Groups in American Society and the Rise of the Young-Old," *Annals of the American Academy of Political and Social Science* 415 (1974): 187.

Chapter 2. Mandatory Retirement and Nonhiring

1. U.S. Department of Labor, *Interim Report to Congress on Age Discrimination in Employment Act Studies, Report to the Congress Required by Section 5 of the Age Discrimination in Employment Act*, prepared for the U.S. Congress by Malcolm H. Morrison and Betty H. Roberts (Washington, D.C.: U.S. Government Printing Office, 1982), 96, 8.

2. David Hackett Fischer, *Growing Old in America* (New York: Oxford University Press, 1977), 43–44.

3. Lawrence M. Friedman, *A History of American Law* (New York: Simon and Schuster, 1973), 188, 432; Mary R. Dearing, *Veterans in Politics: The Story of the G.A.R.* (Westport, Conn.: Greenwood, 1974).

4. Tamara K. Hareven, "The Last Stage: Historical Adulthood and Old Age," in *Adulthood*, ed. Erik H. Erikson (New York: Norton, 1978), 201, 206.

5. Carole Haber, "Mandatory Retirement in Nineteenth-Century America: The Conceptual Basis for a New Work Cycle," *Journal of Social History* 12 (1978): 84.

6. Hareven, "The Last Stage," 208.

7. Cited in New York Legislature, Joint Legislative Committee on Discrimination in Employment of the Middle Aged, *Preliminary Report* (1938), summarized in "Causes of Discrimination against Older Workers," *Monthly Labor Review* 46 (May 1938): 1139.

8. "Finds Employers Favor No Age Bar: Manufacturers' Association Reports 70% of Concerns Questioned Set No Limit; Many Prefer Older Men; Most Frequent Maximum for Hiring Put at 50 Years for Skilled Workers, 45 for Others," *New York Times*, 21 March 1929, 23.

9. USDL, *Age Discrimination in Employment Studies*, 97.

10. Martin B. Tracy, "Flexible Retirement Features Abroad," *Social Security Bulletin* 41 (May 1978): 10, 27.

11. Edwin F. Witte, *Development of the Social Security Act* (Madison: University of Wisconsin Press, 1963), 159.

12. Senate Committee on Finance, *The Social Security Bill,* 74th Cong., 1st sess., 1935, S. Rept. 628, 10.

13. James T. Sykes, "Mandatory Retirement: An Age-Based Policy Outdated," in *Age or Need? Public Policies for Older People,* ed. Bernice L. Neugarten (Beverly Hills: Sage, 1982); Wilma Donahue, Harold L. Orbach, and Otto Pollack, "Retirement: The Emerging Social Pattern," in *Handbook of Social Gerontology: Societal Aspects of Aging,* ed. Clark Tibbitts (Chicago: University of Chicago Press, 1960), 330.

14. Tracy, "Flexible Retirement," 19. Payment ages are one of the tools in using social security changes to manipulate the labor supply and as elements of public policy. See A. Zabalza and D. Piachaud, "Social Security and the Elderly: A Simulation of Policy Changes," *Journal of Public Economics* 16 (1981): 145–69.

15. See J. Douglas Brown, *An American Philosophy of Social Security* (Princeton: Princeton University Press, 1972); Eveline M. Burns, *The American Social Security System* (Boston: Houghton Mifflin, 1949).

16. William Graebner, *A History of Retirement: The Meaning and Function of an American Institution, 1885–1978* (New Haven: Yale University Press, 1980).

17. Fred Cottrell, "The Technological and Societal Basis of Aging," in Tibbitts, *Handbook of Social Gerontology.*

18. Malcolm H. Morrison, "Work and Retirement in an Aging Society," *Daedalus* 115 (Winter 1986): 279 (reprinted in *Our Aging Society: Paradox and Promise,* ed. Alan Pifer and Lydia Bronte [New York: Norton, 1986]).

19. Edward Howard, Nancy Peavy, and Lauren Selden, "Age Discrimination and Mandatory Retirement," in *Economics of Aging: The Future of Retirement,* ed. Malcolm H. Morrison (New York: Van Nostrand Reinhold, 1982), 52.

20. Tracy, "Flexible Retirement," 19.

21. Morrison, "Work and Retirement in an Aging Society," 278.

22. Martin L. Levine, "The Emergence of Special Rights for the Elderly in National Law around the World," in *More to Life: Proceedings of the XI International Conference of Gerontology* (Paris: International Center of Social Gerontology, 1987).

23. U.S. Bureau of the Census, *Current Population Reports,* Special Studies, Series P-23, no. 59 (1976).

24. Matilda White Riley and Anne Foner, *An Inventory of Research Findings,* vol. 1 of *Aging and Society* (New York: Russell Sage, 1968), 42. Moreover, between 1955 and 1975, the fraction of male population aged 55–64 who participated in the labor force steadily dropped, from 9 out of 10 to 3 out of 4. Considering just those 60–64 years of age, the decline in labor-force participation was even more noticeable: from 4 out of 5 in 1955 to 2 out of 3 in 1975. The most dramatic reduction in labor force participation by those 60–64 years of age—from 75% to 65.7%—occurred in the early 1970s. U.S. Bureau of the Census, *Current Population Reports.*

25. Juanita M. Kreps, "Aggregate Income and Labor Force Participation of the Aged," *Law and Contemporary Problems* 27 (1962): 66; Stephen R. McConnell,

"Retirement and Employment," in *Aging: Scientific Perspectives and Social Issues*, 2d ed., ed. Diana S. Woodruff and James E. Birren (Monterey, Calif.: Brooks/Cole, 1983), 335.

26. Philip L. Rones, "Older Men—The Choice between Work and Retirement," *Monthly Labor Review* 101 (November 1978): 3–10.

27. House Select Committee on Aging, *Abolishing Mandatory Retirement*, 97th Cong., 1st sess., 1981, Committee Print, 4.

28. Rose Laub Coser, *The Family: Its Structures and Functions* (New York: St. Martin's, 1974) (the British study); David T. Barker and Robert L. Clark, "Mandatory Retirement and Labor-Force Participation of Respondents in the Retirement History Study," *Social Security Bulletin* 43 (November 1980): 20–29.

29. Donahue, Orbach, and Pollack, "Retirement: The Emerging Social Pattern," 359–60; Rones, "Older Men." See also Lois Farrer Copperman and Frederick D. Keast, *Adjusting to an Older Work Force* (New York: Van Nostrand Reinhold, 1983), 70; R. Clark, *Adjusting Hours to Increase Jobs*, Special Report no. 15 to the National Commission for Manpower Policy (1977); Richard N. Barfield and James Morgan, *Early Retirement: The Decision and the Experience* (Ann Arbor: Survey Research Center, University of Michigan, 1969).

30. House Comm. on Aging, *Abolishing Mandatory Retirement*, 5.

31. Erdman B. Palmore, Bruce M. Burchett, Gerda G. Fillenbaum, Linda K. George, and Laurence M. Wallman, *Retirement: Causes and Consequences* (New York: Springer, 1985), 170–72. Over their lifetimes, men will work a third longer than women (about 39 years to 29), and whites will work longer than minority group members (nearly 7 years longer, for men). These are estimates of work life from birth onward assuming 1979–80 rates hold constant, as prepared by the U.S. Bureau of Labor Statistics. Shirley J. Smith, "Revised Worklife Tables Reflect 1979–80 Experience," *Monthly Labor Review* 108 (August 1985): 23–30.

32. See Lenore E. Bixby, "Retirement Patterns in the United States: Research and Policy Interaction," *Social Security Bulletin* 39 (August 1976): 3–19; Colin D. Campbell and Rosemary G. Campbell, "Conflicting Views on the Effect of Old-Age and Survivors' Insurance on Retirement," *Economic Inquiry* 14 (1976): 369; Robin Jane Walther, "Economics of Aging," in Woodruff and Birren, *Aging*, 370.

33. Gary S. Fields and Olivia S. Mitchell, *Retirement, Pensions, and Social Security*. (Cambridge: MIT Press, 1984).

34. Ibid.; U.S. Senate Special Committee on Aging, *Emerging Options for Work and Retirement Policy: An Analysis of Major Income and Employment Issues with an Agenda for Research Priorities*, 96th Cong., 2d sess., 1980, Committee Print.

35. Fields and Mitchell, *Retirement, Pensions, and Social Security*, 5–6, Table 1.3

36. Barker and Clark, "Mandatory Retirement," 28.

37. U.S. Department of Labor, *The Older American Worker: Age Discrimination in Employment, Report to Congress under Section 715 of Civil Rights Act of 1964* (Washington, D.C.: U.S. Government Printing Office, 1965), 7.

38. Ibid., 6–7, 17.
39. House Comm. on Aging, *Abolishing Mandatory Retirement*, v.
40. USDL, *Age Discrimination in Employment Studies*, 6. Halpern, using data from the National Longitudinal Survey for 1971, reported a similar figure: nearly half of male wage earners worked in jobs with mandatory retirement. Barker and Clark reported that mandatory retirement provisions covered about 2 out of 5 of the cohort of white male wage earners aged 62–63 in 1969. The figure for workers of both sexes was 37% according to Clark, Barker, and Cantrell, and also Burkhauser and Quinn. A variety of studies in the 1960s and '70s of percentage of employees covered by mandatory retirement rules yielded figures of 30%, 41%, 49%, and 61%. See Staff of House Select Committee on Aging, *Mandatory Retirement: The Social and Human Costs of Enforced Idleness*, 95th Cong., 1st sess., 1977, Committee Print; Janice Halpern, "Raising the Mandatory Retirement Age: Its Effect on the Employment of Older Workers," *New England Economic Review*, May–June 1978, 23–35; Barker and Clark, "Mandatory Retirement"; Robert L. Clark, David T. Barker, and Steven R. Cantrell, eds., *Outlawing Age Discrimination: Economic and Institutional Response to the Elimination of Mandatory Retirement*, Final Report to the Administration on Aging under Grant 90-A-1738, September 1979, cited in Fields and Mitchell, *Retirement, Pensions, and Social Security;* Richard V. Burkhauser and Joseph F. Quinn, "Is Mandatory Retirement Overrated? Evidence from the 1970's," *Journal of Human Resources* 18 (1983): 357.
41. Barker and Clark, "Mandatory Retirement," 21, 24.
42. The Canadian *Survey of Retirement* suggests a figure of 8%–10% for those who retired because of compulsory retirement and who were dissatisfied with the timing of their retirement. Statistics Canada, *Survey of Retirement*, Labour Force Supplement (1975). Another study concluded that about 7% of all retired U.S. male workers wanted to work and were able to do so, but were retired and could not find new jobs. James H. Schulz, "The Economics of Mandatory Retirement," *Industrial Gerontology* 1 (Winter 1974): 1–10, 5. A study conducted in the mid-1970s concluded that roughly 6% of men subject to mandatory retirement who were working in 1973 would have remained working in 1975 but for mandatory retirement at 65. Burkhauser and Quinn, "Is Mandatory Retirement Overrated?" Still another study concluded that about one-half of those now retired would have preferred to continue working. Louis Harris and Associates, Inc., *1979 Study of American Attitudes toward Pensions and Retirement: A Nationwide Survey of Employees, Retirees, and Business Leaders: Summary* (New York: Johnson and Higgins, 1979).
43. R. G. Axelbank, "The Position of the Older Worker in the American Labor Force," in *Employment of the Middle-Aged*, ed. Gloria M. Shatto (Springfield, Ill.: C. C. Thomas, 1972).
44. W. W. Daniel, *National Survey of the Unemployed* (London: Political and Economic Planning, 1974). According to U.K. Department of Employment figures, more than half of those over age 55 who were registered as unemployed had been

out of work more than a year, far longer than in other age groups. In the United Kingdom in 1980, Jolly, Creigh, and Mingay surveyed 16,000 job vacancies using national records from the Manpower Services Commission; for 27.5% of the vacancies there were age-related hiring limits, particularly in distributive trades and manufacturing industries. Where there was an age limit, 65% of jobs were closed to all applicants over 40; 76% of professional jobs were closed to those over 50. The British study also found that age is an increasingly important criterion for selecting workers for redundancy. T. Jolly, S. Creigh, and A. Mingay, *Age as a Factor in Employment,* Research Paper no. 11 (London: Department of Economics, 1980), cited in D. R. Davies and Paul R. Sparrow, "Age and Work Behavior," in *Aging and Human Performance,* ed. Neil Charness (New York: John Wiley and Sons, 1985), 299–300.

45. Barker and Clark, "Mandatory Retirement," 22.
46. USDL, *Age Discrimination in Employment Studies,* 101, 102.
47. Ibid.
48. House Select Committee on Aging, *Eliminating Mandatory Retirement,* 99th Cong., 2d sess., 1986, Committee Print, 6.
49. Claude Pepper, "Foreword," in House Comm. on Aging, *Abolishing Mandatory Retirement,* iv.
50. Staff of House Comm. on Aging, *Mandatory Retirement.*
51. Pepper, "Foreword," in House Comm. on Aging, *Abolishing Mandatory Retirement,* iv.
52. Donald O. Cowgill, "The Aging of Populations and Societies," *Annals of the American Academy of Political and Social Science* 415 (1974): 12–13.
53. USDL, *The Older American Worker.*
54. U.S. Bureau of the Census, *Current Population Reports; Hearings on Future Developments in Social Security before the Senate Special Comm. on Aging,* 94th Cong., 1st sess., 19 March 1975; Palmore et al., *Retirement,* 167.
55. William C. Greenough and Francis P. King, *Pension Plans and Public Policy* (New York: Columbia University Press, 1976); Arthur Okun, "Inflation: The Problems and Prospects before Us," in *Inflation: The Problems It Creates and the Policies It Requires,* ed. Arthur Okun, Henry H. Fowler, and Milton Gilbert (New York: New York University Press, 1970).
56. Renegotiation Amendments of 1973, Pub. L. No. 93–66, § 201(a)(1), 87 Stat. 152 (codified as amended at 42 U.S.C.A. § 415 (West Supp. 1987)).
57. Robert N. Butler, *Why Survive? Being Old in America* (New York: Harper and Row, 1975).
58. Karn C. Holden, Daniel Feaster, and Richard Burkhauser, "The Risk and Timing of Poverty after Retirement," reported in *Gerontologist* 26 (1986): 261A.
59. *New York Times,* 28 January 1987, A17, col. 1.
60. "The Retirement Equity Act: Progress toward Private Pension Equity for Women," *NSCLC Washington Weekly,* 7 February 1986, 21–22.
61. The Retirement Equity Act of 1984, Pub. L. No. 98–397, 98 Stat. 1426 (codified as amended at 26 U.S.C.A. §§ 72, 401, *et seq.,* 6057, 6652 (West Supp. 1987)).

62. E.g., Hampton v. Mow Sun Wong, 426 U.S. 88 (1976): A Civil Service Commission regulation that "exclude[s] all noncitizens [including legally admitted resident aliens] from the federal service, . . . broadly denying this class substantial opportunities for employment, . . . deprives its members of an aspect of liberty." Ibid. at 116.

63. Milton L. Barron, *The Aging American: An Introduction to Social Gerontology and Geriatrics* (Westport, Conn.: Greenwood, 1961); Edmund C. Payne, "Depression and Suicide," in *Modern Perspectives in the Psychiatry of Old Age,* ed. John G. Howells (New York: Brunner/Mazel, 1975), 290; G. Streib, "Morale of the Retired," *Social Problems* 3 (1956): 270.

64. *Congressional Record,* 1967, 113:35056 (statement of Sen. Randolph quoting gerontologist Donald P. Kent at August 1964 hearings on Senate Special Committee on Aging).

65. AMA report cited in Senate Committee on Human Resources, *Amending the Age Discrimination in Employment Act Amendments of 1977,* 95th Cong., 1st sess., 12 October 1977, S. Rept. 493, 4; Robert C. Atchley, "Retirement: Leaving the World of Work," *Annals of the American Academy of Political and Social Science* 464 (1982): 120–31.

66. Palmore et al., *Retirement,* 167–68.

67. D. Ekerdt, L. Baden, R. Bosse, and E. Dibbs, "The Effects of Retirement on Physical Health," *American Journal of Public Health* 73 (1983): 779–83.

68. Pepper, "Foreword," in House Comm. on Aging, *Abolishing Mandatory Retirement,* iv–v; see ibid., 5.

69. Senate Comm. on Human Resources, *Amending the Age Discrimination in Employment Act,* 4.

70. Stephen R. McConnell, "Alternative Work Patterns for an Aging Work Force," in *Work and Retirement: Policy Issues,* ed. Pauline K. Ragan (Los Angeles: University of Southern California Press, 1980), 82.

71. William Oriol, "Work and Retirement: Visible Issues at U.N. World Assembly on Aging," *Aging and Work* 7 (1984): 13–20.

72. Louis Harris and Associates, Inc., *Aging in the Eighties: America in Transition,* conducted for the National Council on Aging (Washington, D.C.: National Council on the Aging, 1981), xiv. See also Carolyn E. Usher, "Alternative Work Options for Older Workers, Part I: Employers' Interest," *Aging and Work* 4 (1981): 74–80. Some empirical support for the thesis that employees reject renegotiation is found, however, in a survey of 333 older workers in Los Angeles County, who had a median age of 58 years and a medium income of $31,000. In this study, slightly more than half of those surveyed stated an interest in some form of employment continued beyond the age of normal retirement. Of those, however, only 5% expressed an interest if there were to be a 10% reduction in wages. In this survey, though, the sample was relatively small and unrepresentative, and the survey questions were inartfully drafted as to the nature of a job modification.

73. Harris and Assoc., *Aging in the Eighties,* xiv.

74. Rones, "Older Men—The Choice," 5.

75. Melvin K. Bers, *Union Policy and the Older Worker* (Berkeley: Institute of Industrial Relations, University of California, Berkeley, 1957), 77–79.
76. Harris and Assoc., *Aging in the Eighties*, xv.
77. Palmore et al., *Retirement*, 169.
78. Benson Rosen, Thomas H. Jerdee, and Robert O. Lunn, "Retirement Policies and Management Decisions," *Aging and Work* 3 (1980): 239–46.
79. Copperman and Keast, *Adjusting to an Older Work Force*, chap. 5. See also Geneva Mathiason, *Flexible Retirement: Evolving Policies and Programs for Industry and Labor* (New York: Putnam, 1957).
80. Copperman and Keast, *Adjusting to an Older Work Force*, 144.
81. Senate Special Committee on Aging, *Personnel Practices for an Aging Work Force: Private-Sector Examples*, Information Paper Prepared for Use by the U.S. Senate, 99th Cong., 1st sess., 1985, Committee Print.
82. National Commission for Employment Policy, *Older Worker Employment Comes of Age: Practice and Potential* (Washington, D.C.: U.S. Government Printing Office, 1986).
83. Committee for Economic Development, *Jobs for the Hard-to-Employ: New Directions for Public-Private Partnership: A Statement by the Research and Policy Committee of the Committee for Economic Development* (New York: Committee for Economic Development, 1978), 59–65; see also Committee for Economic Development, *Reforming Retirement Policies: A Statement by the Research and Policy Committee of the Committee for Economic Development* (New York: Committee for Economic Development, 1981), 45–46.
84. M. H. Morrison, *Maximizing Employment Opportunities for the Midlife and Older Worker: The Employer's and Employee's Perspectives, International Forum* (Jerusalem: Brookdale Institute of Gerontology, 1986). See also M. H. Morrison, *The Transition to Retirement* (Washington, D.C.: Bureau of Social Science Research, 1985).
85. Tracy, "Flexible Retirement," 25.
86. G. Crona, "Flexible Retirement: The Case of Sweden," in *Effecting Options for Income and Life Satisfaction: The Norway and Sweden Experience*, cited in Helen Ginsburg, "Flexible and Partial Retirement for Norwegian and Swedish Workers," *Monthly Labor Review* 108 (October 1985): 38.
87. Cited in Ginsburg, "Flexible and Partial Retirement for Norwegian and Swedish Workers," 39, Table 4. See also Martin Tracy, *Retirement Age Practices in Ten Industrial Societies, 1960–1976*, Studies and Research no. 14 (Geneva: International Social Security Association, 1979); Leif Haanes-Olson, "New Retirement Options in Sweden," *Social Security Bulletin* 39 (March 1976): 31.
88. S. Smirnov, "The Employment of Old-Age Pensioners in the USSR," *International Labour Review* 116 (1977): 87–94.
89. Christopher Mackaronis, "Employment 'Exit Incentives' Enter the Courts," *Working Age* (AARP Worker Equity Dept. newsletter) 2 (July/August 1986): 1.
90. "Abbey National Offers Retirement to Over-50's," *The Times* (London), 6 Jan. 1986, 3.

Chapter 3.   Puzzles and Models

1. Meta-analysis is the practice of taking previously performed studies, appropriately combining their data, and drawing conclusions from the combined data.
2. Edmund S. Phelps, *Inflation Policy and Unemployment Theory: The Cost-Benefit Approach to Monetary Planning* (New York: Norton, 1972), 25–26; Phelps, "The Statistical Theory of Racism and Sexism," *American Economic Review* 62 (1972): 659.
3. Gary S. Becker, *The Economics of Discrimination,* 2d ed. (Chicago: University of Chicago Press, 1971).
4. See, e.g., H. Manne, *The Economics of Legal Relationships: Readings in the Theory of Property Rights* (St. Paul: West Publishing Co., 1975); Richard A. Posner, *Economic Analysis of Law,* 2d ed. (Boston: Little, Brown, 1977).
5. See Chapter 7.
6. Edward P. Lazear, "Why Is There Mandatory Retirement?" *Journal of Political Economy* 87 (1979): 1261–84.
7. Sigmund Freud, "Formulations on the Two Principles of Mental Functioning" (1911), in *The Standard Edition of the Complete Psychological Works of Sigmund Freud,* ed. and trans. James Strachey (London: Hogarth Press, 1975), vol. 12; Sigmund Freud, *Beyond the Pleasure Principle* (1920), ibid., vol. 18; Sigmund Freud, *The Ego and the Id* (1923), ibid., vol. 22.

Chapter 4.   Discrimination and Stereotype Theories

1. New York Legislature, Joint Legislative Committee on Discrimination in Employment of the Middle Aged, *Preliminary Report* (1938), summarized in "Causes of Discrimination against Older Workers," *Monthly Labor Review* 46 (May 1938): 1139.
2. G. Boglietti, "Discrimination against Older Workers and the Promotion of Equality and Opportunity," *International Labour Review* 110 (1974): 357–58; Age Discrimination in Employment Act of 1967, §6, Pub. L. No. 90–202, 81 Stat. 602 (1967). Prohibitions of mandatory retirement were added by the Age Discrimination in Employment Act Amendments of 1978, Pub. L. No. 95–256, 92 Stat. 189 (codified as amended at 29 U.S.C.A. §§ 623–34 (West Supp. 1987)).
3. New York Legislature, *Preliminary Report,* 1143, 1139.
4. Ibid. (quoting the committee report).
5. Harland Fox, "Utilization of Older Manpower," *Harvard Business Review* 29 (1951): 45.
6. Beatrice Brower, *Trends in Company Pension Plans,* Studies in Personnel Policy, no. 61 (New York: National Industrial Conference Board, 1944).
7. Fox, "Utilization of Older Manpower," citing J. A. Sheldon, "Medical-Social Aspects of the Aging Process," in *The Aged and Society,* 226.

8. Lloyd G. Reynolds and Joseph Shister, *Job Horizons: A Study of Job Satisfaction and Labor Mobility* (New York: Harper & Brothers, 1949), 71.
9. Fox, "Utilization of Older Manpower."
10. Brower, *Trends in Company Pension Plans,* 10.
11. Because there were no studies of productivity or health done at that time. Carole Haber, "Mandatory Retirement in Nineteenth-Century America: The Conceptual Basis for a New Work Cycle," *Journal of Social History* 12 (1978): 87.
12. New York Legislature, *Preliminary Report,* 1139.

Chapter 5. Macroeconomic Theories

1. Clarence D. Long, *The Labor Force under Changing Income and Employment,* National Bureau of Economic Research, General Series no. 65 (Princeton: Princeton University Press, 1958).
2. Considering overall labor supply and demand, Long found a clear association between reduction in labor-force participation of elderly males and level of unemployment, change in unemployment, and unemployment among different industries. All these findings are consistent with the possibility that elderly men left the labor force because they were discouraged by lack of jobs. He concluded that there is no close relation between labor-force participation by the elderly and general unemployment.

   Long noted the possibility that age-work policies accounted for the declining participation of the elderly in the labor force, but did not regard it as definitively established that age-work policies had become more extensive during the period during which elderly labor-force participation declined. A 1949 study by the National Association of Manufacturers found about the same proportion of firms with nonhiring policies for the elderly as a similar study by the NAM two decades before (1930). Another survey consistent with those findings is Albert J. Abrams, "Barriers to Employment of Older Workers," *Annals of the American Academy of Political and Social Science* 279 (1952): 62. Thus, Long regarded his study as more salient for voluntary withdrawal of the aged from the work force.
3. Long, *The Labor Force,* 167.
4. Robert M. MacDonald, *Mandatory Retirement and the Law* (Washington, D.C.: American Enterprise Institute for Public Policy Research, 1978).
5. A survey of twenty-six large manufacturing companies concluded that some employers hesitated to hire older workers partly in the belief they were less versatile (Dwight L. Palmer and John A. Brownell, "Influence of Age on Employment Opportunities," *Monthly Labor Review* 48 [April 1939]: 765), but that study could not find any general tendency for older workers to be less productive or have more accidents. Presumably, ineffective workers of any age were weeded out. Nor was there widespread prejudice among executives against older workers, based on supposed low productivity or high accident or sickness rates. Thus,

even in 1939, some scholars and executives had concluded that notions about the unproductivity of older workers were unsupported.

6. Ibid.
7. Gene W. Dalton and Paul H. Thompson, "Accelerating Obsolescence of Older Engineers," *Harvard Business Review* 49 (September–October 1971): 57.
8. See Chapter 6, below.
9. Long, *The Labor Force,* 168; see Harland Fox, "Utilization of Older Manpower," *Harvard Business Review* 29 (1951): 44, 51.
10. See H. A. Rusk, "65 Plus No Bar to Congress But End of Line in Industry; Retirement Policies Seen in Need of Revision to Avert National Crisis within 30 Years," *New York Times,* 24 February 1952, 67.
11. U.S. Department of Labor, Bureau of Economic Security, *Older Worker Adjustment to Labor Market Practices: Analysis of Experience in Seven Major Labor Markets* (Washington, D.C.: U.S. Government Printing Office, 1956).
12. Long, *The Labor Force,* 171.
13. Ibid., 268, 179.
14. Erdman Palmore, "When Can Age, Period, and Cohort be Separated?" *Social Forces* 57 (1978): 1.
15. E.g., Abrams, "Barriers"; Margaret S. Gordon, "The Older Worker and Retirement Policies," *Monthly Labor Review* 83 (June 1960): 577; Juanita M. Kreps, "Economics of Retirement," in *Behavior and Adaption in Late Life,* ed. Ewald B. Busse and Eric Pfeiffer (Boston: Little, Brown, 1969), 71.
16. Kreps, "Economics of Retirement," 81.
17. Ibid., 82.
18. Ibid., 81.
19. Juanita M. Kreps, "Aggregate Income and Labor Force Participation of the Aged," *Law and Contemporary Problems* 27 (1962): 62.
20. G. Boglietti, "Discrimination against Older Workers and the Promotion of Equality and Opportunity," *International Labour Review* 110 (1974): 355.
21. Kreps, "Aggregate Income," 62.
22. Sara Leiter, "Hiring Policies, Prejudices, and the Older Worker," *Monthly Labor Review* 88 (August 1965): 968, excerpted from U.S. Department of Labor, *The Older American Worker: Age Discrimination in Employment, Report of Secretary of Labor to Congress under Section 715 of Civil Rights Act of 1964, Research Materials* (Washington, D.C.: U.S. Government Printing Office, 1965).
23. Leiter, "Hiring Policies," 969.
24. Ibid.
25. Ibid., 970.
26. Ibid.
27. Ibid.
28. Ibid.
29. Lois F. Copperman and Frederick D. Keast, *Adjusting to An Older Work Force* (New York: Van Nostrand Reinhold, 1983), 147–48.
30. William Graebner, *A History of Retirement: The Meaning and Function of an American Institution, 1885–1978* (New Haven: Yale University Press, 1980).

31. Robert Clark, Juanita Kreps, and Joseph Spengler, "Economics of Aging: A Survey," *Journal of Economic Literature* 16 (1978): 919.

32. Kreps, "Economics of Retirement," 82–83.

33. Juanita Kreps and Joseph Spengler, "The Leisure Component of Economic Growth," *Technology and the American Economy,* vol. 2, appendix (Washington, D.C.: U.S. Government Printing Office, 1966), 355.

34. Carole Haber, "Mandatory Retirement in Nineteenth-Century America: The Conceptual Basis for A New Work Cycle," *Journal of Social History* 12 (1978): 77.

35. Frank F. Furstenberg, Jr., and Charles A. Thrall, "Counting the Jobless: The Impact of Job Rationing on Measures of Unemployment," *Annals of the American Academy of Political and Social Science* 418 (1975): 45–59.

36. Edmund S. Phelps, "The Statistical Theory of Racism and Sexism," *American Economic Review* 62 (1972): 659–61.

37. Cf. Edward Howard, Nancy Peavy, and Lauren Selden, "Age Discrimination and Mandatory Retirement," in *Economics of Aging: The Future of Retirement,* ed. Malcolm H. Morrison (New York: Van Nostrand Reinhold, 1982), 217.

38. Furstenberg and Thrall, "Counting the Jobless," 59.

Chapter 6. The Age-Bonus Theory

1. Edward P. Lazear, "Why Is There Mandatory Retirement?" *Journal of Political Economy* 87 (1979): 1261–84.

2. Robert E. Hall, "Employment Fluctuations and Wage Rigidity," *Brookings Papers on Economic Activity,* 1980, 91. But cf. Benjamin Klein, "Contract Costs and Administered Prices: An Economic Theory of Rigid Wages," *American Economic Association: Papers and Proceedings* 74 (May 1984): 332–38 (risk-neutral terms keep open an escape hatch so workers can be terminated if necessary).

3. See works cited by Edward P. Lazear, "Incentives and Wage Rigidity," *American Economic Association: Papers and Proceedings* 74 (May 1984): 341.

4. D. T. Hall, *Careers in Organizations* (Pacific Palisades, Calif.: Goodyear, 1976).

5. Harris Shrank and Joan Waring, "Aging and Work Organizations," in *Leading Edges: Recent Research In Psychosocial Aging,* ed. Beth B. Hess and Kathleen Bond (Washington, D.C.: U.S. Department of Health and Human Services, Public Health Service, National Institutes of Health, U.S. Government Printing Office, 1981), 91.

6. James E. Rosenbaum, "Organizational Career Mobility: Promotion Chances in a Corporation during Periods of Growth and Contraction," *American Journal of Sociology* 85 (1979): 21; idem, "Tournament Mobility: Career Patterns in a Corporation," *Administrative Science Quarterly* 24 (1979): 220.

7. E.g., Mark E. Schaefer, Fred A. Massey, and Roger H. Hermanson, "The Peter Principle Revisited," *Across the Board* 17 (July 1980): 3.

8. Schrank and Waring, "Aging and Work Organizations."

9. Lazear, "Why Is There Mandatory Retirement?"

10. Herbert A. Simon, *Administrative Behavior: A Study of Decision-Making Processes in Administrative Organization* (New York: Free Press, 1976); Richard Craswell, personal communication, 15 February 1984.

11. Lazear, "Incentives," 340.

12. Sidford Brown, personal communication, 13 June 1982.

13. John Lapp, "An Economic Model of Early Retirement," in *Outlawing Age Discrimination: Economic and Institutional Response to the Elimination of Mandatory Retirement,* ed. Robert L. Clark, David T. Barker, and Steven R. Cantrell, Final Report to the Administration on Aging under Grant 90-A-1738, January 1980, 39–62.

14. John Rawls, *A Theory of Justice* (Cambridge: Belknap Press of Harvard University Press, 1971), sec. 24.

15. Lazear, "Why Is There Mandatory Retirement?"

16. David T. Barker, "Mandatory Retirement: Theories and Evidence" (Unpublished manuscript, George Fox College, 16 July 1981).

17. Robert J. Flanagan, "Implicit Contracts, Explicit Contracts, and Wages," *American Economic Association: Papers and Proceedings* 74 (May 1984): 345–349.

18. Martin Neil Baily, "Wages and Unemployment under Uncertain Demand," *Review of Economic Studies* 41 (1974): 37.

19. Michael L. Wachter and Oliver E. Williamson, "Obligational Markets and the Mechanics of Inflation," *Bell Journal of Economics* 9 (1978): 549–71.

20. Edward P. Lazear, "Agency, Earnings Profiles, Productivity, and Hours Restrictions," *American Economic Review* 71 (1981): 606–20.

21. Margaret S. Gordon, "The Older Worker and Retirement Policies," *Monthly Labor Review* 83 (June 1960): 579.

22. Dorothy R. Kittner, "Forced Retirement: How Common Is It?" *Monthly Labor Review* 100 (December 1977): 60–61.

23. Thomas C. Schelling, "Self-Command in Practice, in Policy, and in a Theory of Rational Choice," *American Economic Association: Papers and Proceedings* 74 (May 1984): 1–11.

24. Massachusetts Bd. of Retirement v. Murgia, 427 U.S. 307 (1976); Vance v. Bradley, 440 U.S. 93 (1979).

25. Martin Levine, "Four Models for Age/Work Policy Research," *Gerontologist* 20 (1980): 561.

26. Evan K. Rowe and Thomas H. Paine, "Pension Plans under Collective Bargaining Agreements: Part II," *Monthly Labor Review* 76 (May 1953): 484; see also Helen Baker, *Retirement Procedures under Compulsory and Flexible Retirement* (Princeton: Princeton University Industrial Relations Section, 1952).

27. Richard M. Cohn, "Contract and Discrimination in Retirement Policy: An Evaluation of Lazear's 'Mandatory Retirement'" (n.p., 1981): 8.

28. Juanita M. Kreps, "A Case Study of Variables in Retirement Policy," *Monthly Labor Review* 84 (June 1961): 587, 590.

29. U.S. Department of Labor, *The Older American Worker: Age Discrimination in Employment, Report of Secretary of Labor to Congress under Section 715 of Civil Rights Act of 1964, Research Materials* (Washington, D.C.: U.S. Government Printing Office, 1965), table 4.
30. Geoffrey Carliner, "The Wages of Older Men," *Journal of Human Resources* 17 (1982): 25.
31. Lazear, "Why Is There Mandatory Retirement?"
32. E. H. Boyle, E. J. Mutran, and C. W. Mueller, "The Influence of Labor Market Characteristics on Age Discrimination in Wages," reported in *Gerontologist* 26 (1986): 261A.

Chapter 7. The Union Choice Theory

1. Margaret S. Gordon, "The Older Worker and Retirement Policies," *Monthly Labor Review* 83 (June 1960): 577–85; Juanita M. Kreps, "A Case Study of Variables in Retirement Policy," *Monthly Labor Review* 84 (June 1961): 587.
2. Richard M. Cohn, "Contract and Discrimination in Retirement Policy: An Evaluation of Lazear's 'Mandatory Retirement'" (n.p., 1981).
3. Ibid., table 2.
4. James J. Strnad, personal communication, 7 September 1982.
5. U.S. Department of Labor, *Interim Report to Congress on Age Discrimination in Employment Act Studies: Report to the Congress Required by Section 5 of the Age Discrimination in Employment Act*, prepared by Malcolm H. Morrison and Betty H. Roberts (Washington, D.C.: U.S. Government Printing Office, 1982), 96–97.
6. Richard N. Barfield and James Morgan, *Early Retirement: The Decision and the Experience* (Ann Arbor: Survey Research Center, University of Michigan, 1969), 166; also see Juanita M. Kreps, "Economics of Retirement," in *Behavior and Adaption in Late Life*, ed. Ewald B. Busse and Eric Pfeiffer (Boston: Little, Brown, 1969), 81–82.
7. Ewan Clague, Balraj Palli, and Leo Kramer, *The Aging Worker and the Union* (New York: Praeger, 1971).
8. Evan K. Rowe and Thomas H. Paine, "Pension Plans under Collective Bargaining Agreements: Part II," *Monthly Labor Review* 76 (May 1953): 484.
9. Cohn, "Contract and Discrimination," table 2.
10. Louis Harris and Associates, Inc., *Aging in the Eighties: America in Transition* (Washington, D.C.: National Council on the Aging, 1981), xiii.
11. Anne Foner and Karen Schwab, *Aging and Retirement* (Monterey, Calif.: Brooks/Cole, 1981), 28.
12. Cohn, "Contract and Discrimination," table 2.
13. Ibid., 10, 21, n. 11.
14. U.S. Commissioner of Labor, *Twenty-Third Annual Report (1908): Workman's Insurance and Benefit Funds in the United States* (Washington, D.C.: U.S. Government Printing Office, 1909), 33.

15. Carole Haber, "Mandatory Retirement in Nineteenth-Century America: The Conceptual Basis for a New Work Cycle," *Journal of Social History* 12 (1978): 77–96.
16. Albert J. Abrams, "Barriers to Employment of Older Workers," *Annals of the American Academy of Political and Social Science* 279 (1952): 62–71.
17. Inland Steel Co., 77 N.L.R.B. 1 (1948), *enforced sub nom.* Inland Steel Co. v. N.L.R.B., 170 F.2d 247 (7th Cir. 1948), *cert. denied on this issue,* 366 U.S. 960 (1949). See Cleveland Board of Education v. LaFleur, 414 U.S. 623, 657 (1974) (dissenting opinion).
18. H. M. Douty, *The Wage Bargain and the Labor Market* (Baltimore: Johns Hopkins University Press, 1980), 7–8.
19. Gordon, "The Older Worker and Retirement Policies"; Clague, Palli, and Kramer, *The Aging Worker and the Union,* 128.
20. Gordon, "The Older Worker and Retirement Policies."
21. Rowe and Paine, "Pension Plans"; see also Samuel Barkin, "Should There Be a Fixed Retirement Age? Organized Labor Says No," in *Social Contribution by the Aging,* ed. Clark Tibbitts (Philadelphia: American Academy of Political and Social Science, 1952).
22. Clague, Palli, and Kramer, *The Aging Worker and the Union,* 19; Dorothy R. Kittner, "Forced Retirement: How Common Is It?" *Monthly Labor Review* 100 (December 1971): 60–61.
23. Morley Gunderson and James E. Pesando, "Eliminating Mandatory Retirement: Economics and Human Rights," *Canadian Public Policy—Analyse de Politiques* 6 (1980): 352.
24. Ibid., 358, 359.
25. Ibid., 356, 358.
26. Ibid., 358, n. 7.
27. Ibid., 357, n. 6.

Chapter 8. Statistical Discrimination Theories

1. Lester C. Thurow, *Generating Inequality: Mechanisms of Distribution in the U.S. Economy* (New York: Basic Books, 1975); Edmund S. Phelps, *Inflation Policy and Unemployment Theory: The Cost-Benefit Approach to Monetary Planning* (New York: Norton, 1972); Edmund S. Phelps, "The Statistical Theory of Racism and Sexism," *American Economic Review* 62 (1972): 659–61; Kenneth Arrow, "Models of Job Discrimination" and "Some Mathematical Models of Race in the Labor Market," in *Racial Discrimination in Economic Life,* ed. Anthony H. Pascal (Lexington, Mass.: Heath, 1972).
2. T. Ramm, Introduction, in *Discrimination in Employment: A Study of Six Countries by the Comparative Labour Law Group,* ed. F. Schmidt (Stockholm: Almquist & Witsell, 1978), 118.
3. Gary S. Becker, *Human Capital and the Personal Distribution of Income: An Analytical Approach* (Ann Arbor: University of Michigan Institute of Public Ad-

ministration, 1967); Richard M. Cohn, "Quantitative Evidence of Age Discrimination: Some Theoretical Issues and Their Consequences," *Aging and Work* 3 (1980): 149.

4. Dennis J. Aigner and Glen G. Cain, "Statistical Theories of Discrimination in Labor Markets," *Industrial and Labor Relations Review* 30 (1977): 175–87.

5. Richard A. Posner, *The Economics of Justice* (Cambridge: Harvard University Press, 1981); idem, "The De Funis Case and the Constitutionality of Preferential Treatment of Racial Minorities," *Supreme Court Review,* 1974, 1.

6. Idem, *Economic Analysis of Law,* 2d ed. (Boston: Little, Brown, 1977), 368.

7. Thurow, *Generating Inequality,* 172.

8. Ibid., 170–77.

9. Cf. Douglas Laycock and Teresa A. Sullivan, "Sex Discrimination as 'Actuarial Equality': A Rejoinder to Kimball," *American Bar Foundation Research Journal,* 1981, 221–28.

10. 29 U.S.C.A. § 623(f)(1) (West Supp. 1987). See also H. R. 5310, 98th Cong., 2d sess. (1984), the Age Discrimination in Employment Act Public Safety Officers Amendments of 1984, which proposed excluding state and local government police and fire departments from ADEA protections. Cf. Western Air Lines v. Criswell, 472 U.S. 400 (1985). Such employees received temporary exclusion from the uncapping of the age limits enacted by the 1986 ADEA Amendment.

11. Richard N. Barfield and James Morgan, *Early Retirement: The Decision and the Experience* (Ann Arbor: Survey Research Center, University of Michigan, 1969). See also Chapter 2, above.

12. Margaret S. Gordon, "The Older Worker and Retirement Policies," *Monthly Labor Review* 83 (June 1960): 577–85.

13. Philip L. Rones, "The Retirement Decision: A Question of Opportunity?" *Monthly Labor Review* 103 (November 1980): 14–17.

14. Richard M. Cohn, "Contract and Discrimination in Retirement Policy: An Evaluation of Lazear's 'Mandatory Retirement' " (n.p., 1981).

15. Michael J. Boskin, *Too Many Promises: The Uncertain Future of Social Security,* Twentieth-Century Fund Report (Homestead, Ill.: Dow Jones-Irwin, 1986).

16. Keith J. Crocker and Arthur Snow, "The Efficiency Effects of Categorical Discrimination in the Insurance Industry," *Journal of Political Economy* 94 (April 1986): 321–44.

17. Michael Hoy, "Categorizing Risks in the Insurance Industry," *Quarterly Journal of Economics* 97 (May 1982): 321–36.

18. Crocker and Snow, "The Efficiency Effects of Categorical Discrimination," 338.

Chapter 9. Sociological Theories

1. David Hackett Fischer, *Growing Old in America* (New York: Oxford University Press, 1977).

2. Increase Mather, *Two Discourses Shewing, I, That The Lord's Ears are Open to the Prayers of the Righteous, and II, the Dignity and Duty of Aged Servants of*

the Lord (Boston: B. Green for Daniel Henchman, 1716), 63, cited in Fischer, *Growing Old in America,* 37–38.

3. W. Andrew Achenbaum, *Old Age in the New Land* (Baltimore: Johns Hopkins University Press, 1978): idem, "The Obsolescence of Old Age in America, 1865–1914," *Journal of Social History* 8 (1974): 48.

4. See "Growing Old: An Exchange," *New York Review of Books,* 15 September 1977, 47, 48, and works cited in Carole Haber, *Beyond Sixty-Five: The Dilemma of Old Age in America's Past* (New York: Cambridge University Press, 1983), 172.

5. Jane Range and Maris A. Vinovskis, "Images of Elderly in Popular Magazines: A Content Analysis of Littell's *Living Age,* 1845–1882," *Social Science History* 5 (1981): 123.

6. Haber, *Beyond Sixty-Five,* 172–73.

7. Ibid., 174; Carole Haber, "Mandatory Retirement in Nineteenth-Century America: The Conceptual Basis of a New Work Cycle," *Journal of Social History* 12 (1978): 77; William Graebner, *A History of Mandatory Retirement: The Meaning and Function of an American Institution, 1885–1978* (New Haven: Yale University Press, 1980); Gail Buchwalter King and Peter N. Stearns, "The Retirement Experience as a Policy Factor: An Applied History Approach," *Journal of Social History* 14 (1981): 589–625.

8. See Donald O. Cowgill and Lowell D. Holmes, *Aging and Modernization* (New York: Appleton-Century-Crofts, 1972); W. Andrew Achenbaum and Peter N. Stearns, "Old Age and Modernization," *Gerontologist* 18 (1978): 307; Erdman Palmore and Kenneth Manton, "Modernization and the Status of the Aged: International Correlations," *Journal of Gerontology* 29 (1974): 205–10.

9. Jill S. Quadagno, *Aging in Early Industrial Society: Work, Family, and Social Policy in Nineteenth-Century England* (New York: Academic Press, 1980), 3.

10. Ernest Watson Burgess, *Aging in Western Societies* (Chicago: University of Chicago Press, 1960).

11. Donald O. Cowgill, "The Aging of Populations and Societies," *Annals of the American Academy of Political and Social Science* 415 (1974): 1–18; Donald O. Cowgill, "Aging and Modernization: A Revision of the Theory," in *Late Life: Communities and Environmental Policy,* ed. Jaber F. Gubrium (Springfield, Ill.: C. C. Thomas, 1974), 123–46; see also Cowgill and Holmes, *Aging and Modernization.*

12. Cowgill, "Aging and Modernization: A Revision of the Theory," 123.

13. Quadagno, *Aging in Early Industrial Society,* 7.

14. See Fischer, *Growing Old in America;* Achenbaum, *Old Age in the New Land;* Haber, "Mandatory Retirement"; and Graebner, *History of Retirement.*

15. Robert C. Atchley, "Retirement as a Social Institution," *Annual Review of Sociology* 8 (1982): 263.

16. Matilda Riley, Marilyn Johnson, and Anne Foner, *A Sociology of Age Stratification,* vol. 3. of *Aging and Society* (New York: Russell Sage Foundation, 1972).

17. Atchley, "Retirement as a Social Institution," 279.

18. M. Elaine Cumming, "New Thoughts on the Theory of Disengagement," in *New Thoughts on Old Age,* ed. Robert Kastenbaum (New York: Springer, 1964), 11.

19. U.S. Department of Labor, *Interim Report to Congress on Age Discrimination in Employment Act Studies: Report to the Congress Required by Section 5 of the Age Discrimination in Employment Act,* prepared by Malcolm H. Morrison and Betty H. Roberts (Washington, D.C.: U.S. Government Printing Office, 1982), 97.

20. Fischer, *Growing Old in America,* 26–76.

21. James J. Dowd, "Aging as Exchange: A Preface to Theory," *Journal of Gerontology* 30 (1975): 584; idem, "Exchange Rates and Old People," *Journal of Gerontology* 35 (1980): 596.

22. Atchley, "Retirement as a Social Institution."

23. Ibid., 277, citing Achenbaum, *Old Age in the New Land.*

24. Ibid., 268, citing Haber, "Mandatory Retirement."

25. Ibid., 274.

26. Malcolm H. Morrison, "Work and Retirement in an Aging Society," *Daedalus* 115 (Winter 1986): 273 (reprinted in *Our Aging Society: Paradox and Promise,* ed. Alan Pifer and Lydia Bronte [New York: Norton, 1986]).

27. Ibid., 275.

28. Ibid., 276.

29. Ibid.

30. Ibid., 277.

31. Ibid.

32. Ibid., 272.

33. Quadagno, *Aging in Early Industrial Society,* 150.

34. Census of England and Wales (1911), 146, quoted in Quadagno, *Aging in Early Industrial Society,* 151.

35. Quoted in G. B. Morrison, "Age and Unemployment," *Journal of the Statistical Society,* July 1911, 865, quoted in Quadagno, *Aging in Early Industrial Society,* 149–50.

36. Quadagno, *Aging in Early Industrial Society,* 167–68.

37. See Lord George Hamilton, "A Statistical Survey of the Problems of Pauperism," *Journal of the Statistical Society* 74 (December 1910–11): 1.

38. Quadagno, *Aging in Early Industrial Society,* 140.

39. Royal Commission on the Aged Poor, *Minutes of Evidence,* 14 (1895): 910, quoted in Quadagno, *Aging in Early Industrial Society,* 157.

40. Royal Commission on the Aged Poor, *Report,* 14 (1895): 797, quoted in Quadagno, *Aging in Early Industrial Society,* 141.

41. Royal Commission on the Aged Poor, *Report,* 14 (1895): 816, quoted in Quadagno, *Aging in Early Industrial Society,* 140.

Chapter 10. Histories of Retirement

1. Carole Haber, *Beyond Sixty-Five* (New York: Cambridge University Press, 1983), ch. 6; idem, "Mandatory Retirement in Nineteenth-Century America: The Conceptual Basis of a New Work Cycle," *Journal of Social History* 12 (1978);

William Graebner, *A History of Retirement: The Meaning and Function of an American Institution, 1885–1978* (New Haven: Yale University Press, 1980).

2. Haber, "Mandatory Retirement," 78.
3. David Hackett Fischer, *Growing Old in America* (New York: Oxford University Press, 1977), 43–44, 54–55.
4. Ibid., 165–66.
5. Haber, "Mandatory Retirement," 85.
6. Ibid., 86–87.
7. Robert C. Atchley, *The Sociology of Retirement* (Cambridge, Mass.: Schenkman, 1976), 13.
8. Haber, "Mandatory Retirement," 89.
9. Haber, *Beyond Sixty-Five,* chs. 6–7.
10. Ibid., 78–79.
11. Graebner, *History of Retirement,* 18, n. 1.
12. Ibid., 226.
13. Ibid., 18, n. 1.
14. Ibid., 18; 13, 53, 163, 263.
15. Ibid., 24–27.
16. Ibid., 207–10.
17. Ibid., 27–45.
18. Ibid., 51. The survey was reported in "Finds Employers Favor No Age Bar; Manufacturers' Association Reports 70% of Concerns Questioned Set No Limit," *New York Times,* 21 March 1929, p. 23, col. 4.
19. Graebner, *History of Retirement,* 26.
20. E.g., House Select Committee on Aging, *Retirement Age Policies: Hearings before the Select Committee on Aging, House of Representatives,* 95th Cong., 1st sess., 16 March 1977, 2:49–50; also ibid., 48, 69, 87, 91, 96. Graebner, *History of Retirement,* 251–52.
21. Graebner, *History of Retirement,* 263, 265.
22. Ibid., 11, 13, 53, 253. See House Committee on Education and Labor, *Age Discrimination in Employment Act Amendments of 1977, Report to Accompany H.R. 5385,* 95th Cong., 1st sess., 1977, H. Rept. 527.
23. Graebner, *History of Retirement,* 264, 16, 266.
24. Ibid., 167.
25. Ibid., 226.
26. Ibid., 252; Subcommittee on Labor of the Senate Committee on Human Resources, *Age Discrimination in Employment Amendments of 1977: Hearings on S. 1784, To Amend the Age Discrimination in Employment Act of 1967,* 95th Cong., 1st sess., 26 and 27 July 1977, 122–32; House Comm. on Aging, *Retirement Age Policies,* 95th Cong., 1:26, 2:75–76.
27. Graebner, *History of Retirement,* 106, 167.
28. Ibid., 237, 247.
29. Subcommittee on Labor, *Age Discrimination in Employment Amendments of 1977,* 1.

30. Graebner, *History of Retirement,* 27–35.
31. James E. Birren and Wendy Loucks, "Age-Related Change and the Individual," *Chicago-Kent Law Review* 57 (1981): 833.
32. See the Age Discrimination in Employment Act Amendments of 1986, Pub. L. No. 99-592, 100 Stat. 3342, 29 U.S.C.A. §§ 622–24, 630–31 (West Supp. 1987).
33. Graebner, *History of Retirement,* 254–66.
34. The characteristics are set out in Chapter 3, above.
35. Graebner, *History of Retirement,* 267–69.
36. Ibid., 251.
37. Ibid., 207.
38. National Recovery Administration, *What the Blue Eagle Means to You and How You Can Get It* (Washington, D.C.: U.S. Government Printing Office, 1933), 20.
39. Railroad Retirement Act of 1934, Act of 27 June 1934, ch. 868, §§ 1–10, 418 Stat. 1283 to 1289, 45 U.S. Code §§ 201–14 (§§ 201–8 and §§ 210–14 declared unconstitutional in Railroad Retirement Bd. v. Alton R.R., 295 U.S. 330 (1935), § 209 repealed by Act of 6 September 1966, Pub. L. 89–554, § 8(a), 80 Stat. 632, 649).
40. Railroad Retirement Bd. v. Alton R.R., 295 U.S. 330 (1935); Graebner, *History of Retirement,* 161.

Chapter 11.   The Labor Department's Theories

1. U.S. Department of Labor, *Interim Report to Congress on Age Discrimination in Employment Act Studies, Report to the Congress Required by Section 5 of the Age Discrimination in Employment Act,* prepared for the U.S. Congress by Malcolm H. Morrison and Betty H. Roberts (Washington, D.C.: U.S. Government Printing Office, 1982), 96. The report first was published as a committee print of the House Select Committee on Aging, *Abolishing Mandatory Retirement,* 97th Cong., 1st sess., 1981, Committee Print; when references to the report use the pagination of the Congressional publication, the Committee Print title is used. The shorter form is U.S. Department of Labor, *Final Report to Congress on Age Discrimination in Employment Act Studies* (Washington, D.C.: U.S. Department of Labor, 1981) (submitted to Congress in 1982).
2. Malcolm H. Morrison, "Work and Retirement in an Aging Society," *Daedalus* 115 (Winter 1986): 269–83 (reprinted in *Our Aging Society: Paradox and Promise,* ed. Alan Pifer and Lydia Bronte [New York: Norton, 1986]).
3. USDL, *Age Discrimination in Employment Studies,* 96.
4. Cf. "Early History of Age Discrimination in Employment," ibid., 7–9 with "The Development of Mandatory Retirement Policies," ibid., 96–99.
5. House Comm. on Aging, *Abolishing Mandatory Retirement,* 49.
6. USDL, *Age Discrimination in Employment Studies,* 97.
7. John W. McConnell and John J. Corson, *The Economic Needs of Older People* (Baltimore: Lord Baltimore Press, 1956).

8. USDL, *Age Discrimination in Employment Studies*, 97.
9. Ibid., 102.
10. Ibid., 98.
11. Ibid., 102.
12. This explanation was independently developed by Sidford Brown. See Chapter 6, above.
13. USDL, *Age Discrimination in Employment Studies*, 100.
14. Ibid., 101.
15. Ibid., 21.
16. Ibid., 62.
17. Ibid., 85, table 20.
18. Ibid., 62, 43.
19. Ibid., 35.
20. Ibid., 64.

Chapter 12. What Is Aging?

1. Vance v. Bradley, 440 U.S. 93, 112 (1979).
2. Leonard Hayflick, "The Cell Biology of Human Aging," *Scientific American* 242 (January 1980): 58, 61; see generally George A. Sacher, "Theory in Gerontology, Part 1," *Annual Review of Gerontology and Geriatrics* 1 (1980): 3.
3. Richard S. Cutler, "Life-Span Extension," in *Aging: Biology and Behavior,* ed. James L. McGaugh and Sara B. Kiesler (New York: Academic Press, 1981), 37. This theory fits into several of the following ones and is closely correlated to "Hayflick's limit," discussed in the following note.
4. See generally Leonard Hayflick, "Cell Aging," *Annual Review of Gerontology and Geriatrics* 1 (1980): 26. The most interesting finding is that cells removed from an animal and maintained in tissue culture will divide a fairly constant number of times and then stop. This number, known as "Hayflick's limit," remains the same regardless of freezing and thawing and reculturing later. For human cells, the maximum number of divisions appears to be fifty, give or take ten. Thus, there are fewer possible divisions remaining for cells taken from older individuals. George M. Martin, "A Genetic and Evolutionary Perspective on Aging and Longevity," in *Perspectives on Aging: Exploding the Myths,* ed. Priscilla W. Johnson (Cambridge: Ballinger, 1981), 29.
5. Leonard Hayflick, "The Cell Biology of Human Aging," *New England Journal of Medicine* 295 (1976): 1302. These errors may be in any of several areas. They may manifest themselves in the replication of DNA, the cell's genetic blueprint for all of its functions. At first, errors are so few that the cell may continue to function normally, but as the errors are compounded, cell functioning becomes less smooth and eventually comes to a halt. As a corollary, the errors may occur in the synthesis of proteins, the catalysts that actually carry out the instructions of the DNA. As greater portions of the proteins become changed, they lose their effectiveness, and cell functioning is thus impaired. The focus of the errors may

also be in the translation of RNA, the intermediary between DNA and proteins; the result is the same. Gary Lynch and Sara Gerling, "Aging and Brain Plasticity," in McGaugh and Kiesler, *Aging: Biology and Behavior,* 203. Minturn Wright suggests that we bear in mind that while these "errors" are simply random changes, the cells in which they occur are in fairly good condition to begin with, so probability dictates that random changes are much more likely to be deleterious than beneficial (personal communication, May 1986).

The observation that many portions of cellular DNA are merely copies of other portions has led to the formulation of the theory that cells are "prepared" to deal with errors—that they have backup copies. As further changes accumulate, these copies are used up, and the reserves are slowly depleted to the point that important information is lost. Margaret H. Huyck and William J. Hoyer, *Adult Development and Aging* (Belmont, Calif.: Wadsworth, 1982), 83; Hayflick, "Cell Aging," 64–65. As a result, the "redundancy" of DNA buys time by postponing the day of cellular breakdown.

6. Huyck and Hoyer, *Adult Development.* Research has suggested that, in a variety of mammals, longevity is inversely proportional to the speed of repair of damage caused by ultraviolet light. Ronald Wilson Hart and Richard Burton Setlow, "Correlations between Deoxyribonucleic Acid Excision-Repair and Life-Span in a Number of Mammalian Species," *Proceedings of the National Academy of Sciences* 71 (1974): 2169.

7. The recent research is by Roy Walford, as reported by Erik Eckholm, *New York Times,* 10 June 1986, p. C3.

8. Cutler, "Life-Span Extension," 37–38.

9. Hayflick, "Cell Aging," 64–65. This would presumably be for evolutionary reasons related to sexual reproduction. Organisms that multiply by dividing cease to exist as they were before dividing, but they live on in their descendants. Sexually reproducing organisms remain after they reproduce, but they eventually die, making room for their offspring. Indeed, some organisms reproduce only once and die immediately thereafter, a phenomenon known as semelparity.

10. Of particular interest to researchers is the buildup of lipofuscins, oxidized, highly insoluble golden-brown pigments which collect in cells and their constituent organelles throughout life, presumably as metabolic by-products. Martin, "Genetic and Evolutionary Perspective," 175. See also Paul Denny, "The Biological Basis of Aging," in *Aging: Scientific Perspectives and Social Issues,* 2d ed., ed. Diana S. Woodruff and James E. Birren (Monterey, Calif.: Brooks/Cole, 1983), 226.

11. Martin, "Genetic and Evolutionary Perspective," 183; Samuel Goldstein and William Reichel, "Physiological and Biological Aspects of Aging," in *Clinical Aspects of Aging,* ed. William Reichel (Baltimore: Williams and Wilkins, 1978), 431.

12. Even seemingly small changes in temperature, if maintained, can affect lifespan. Huyck and Hoyer, *Adult Development,* 87.

13. E.g., Gregory W. Siskind and Marc E. Weksler, "The Effect of Aging on the

Immune Response," *Annual Review of Gerontology and Geriatrics* 3 (1982): 3; Cutler, "Life-Span Extensions," 58; Robert N. Butler, "Overview on Aging: Some Biomedical, Social, and Behavioral Perspectives," in McGaugh and Kiesler, *Aging: Biology and Behavior,* 1.

14. J. D. Emerson and G. M. Emerson, "Is Aging an Autoimmune Disease? Failure to Decrease Lifespan of the Female Rat by Long-Term Intermittent Adjuvant Administration," in *Aging,* ed. Geraldine M. Emerson (Stroudsberg, Pa.: Dowden, Hutchinson, and Ross, 1977), 312, reprinted from *Alabama Journal of Medical Science* 10 (1973): 281.

15. Lynch and Gerling, "Aging and Brain Plasticity," 207.

16. Eric Eckholm, *New York Times,* 10 June 1986, p. C1.

17. Nathan W. Shock, Richard C. Greulich, Reubin Andres, David Arenberg, Paul T. Costa, Jr., Edward G. Lakatta, and Jordan D. Tobin, *Normal Human Aging: The Baltimore Longitudinal Study of Aging,* NIH Publication 84-2450 (Washington, D.C.: U.S. Government Printing Office, 1984), 207. See also John Morrow and Charles Garner, "An Evaluation of Some Theories of the Mechanism of Aging," *Gerontology* 25 (1979): 136.

18. Cutler, "Life-Span Extension," 32–33.

19. E.g., remarks of Dr. Allan Goldstein, quoted in Ellen Hume, "Science Taps Fountain of Aging Mystery," *Los Angeles Times,* 27 July 1982, sec. I, p. 1; Ben Sherwood, "Berle's New Act: Longevity Research," *Los Angeles Times,* 7 September 1982, sec. V, p. 1; *Newsweek,* 1 November 1982, p. 57.

20. Edward J. Masoro, "Nutritional Intervention in the Aging Process," in *Perspectives on Aging: Exploding The Myths,* ed. Priscilla W. Johnson (Cambridge: Ballinger, 1981), 190–91.

21. Shock et al., *Normal Human Aging.*

22. Paul T. Costa and Robert R. McCrae, "An Approach to the Attribution of Aging, Period, and Cohort Effects," *Psychological Bulletin* 92 (1982): 238–50.

23. E.g., James F. Fries and Lawrence M. Crapo, *Vitality and Aging: Implications of the Rectangular Curve* (San Francisco: Freeman, 1981).

Chapter 13. The Productivity of the Older Worker

1. Robert C. Atchley, *The Sociology of Retirement* (Cambridge, Mass.: Schenkman, 1976), 13.

2. Mildred Doering, Susan R. Rhodes, and Michael Schuster, *The Aging Worker: Research and Recommendations* (Beverly Hills: Sage, 1983); Diana S. Woodruff and James E. Birren, eds., *Aging: Scientific Perspectives and Social Issues,* 2d ed. (Monterey, Calif.: Brooks/Cole, 1983); D. Roy Davies and Paul R. Sparrow, "Age and Work Behavior," in *Aging and Human Performance,* ed. Neil Charness (New York: John Wiley and Sons, 1985).

3. Doering, Rhodes, and Schuster, *The Aging Worker,* 64.

4. U.S. Department of Labor, *The Older American Worker: Age Discrimination in Employment, Report to Congress under Section 715 of Civil Rights Act of 1964* (Washington, D.C.: U.S. Government Printing Office, 1965), 8, 9.

5. Matilda W. Riley and Anne Foner, *An Inventory of Research Findings,* vol. 1 of *Aging and Society* (New York: Russell Sage, 1968).

6. International Labor Organization, *Human Resources Development: Vocational Guidance and Vocational Training,* Report VIII (2), International Labor Conference, 59th Session, 1974, 50, quoted in G. Boglietti, "Discrimination against Older Workers and the Promotion of Equality and Opportunity," *International Labour Review* 110 (1974): 356, n. 3.

7. Senate Committee on Human Resources, *Amending the Age Discrimination in Employment Act Amendments of 1977: Report to Accompany H.R. 5383,* 95th Cong., 1st sess., 12 October 1977, S. Rept. 493.

8. Doering, Rhodes, and Schuster, *The Aging Worker,* 80.

9. Ibid., 80–81.

10. Dorothy Fleisher and Barbara H. Kaplan, "Characteristics of Older Workers: Implications for Restructuring Work," in *Work and Retirement: Policy Issues,* ed. Pauline K. Ragan (Los Angeles: University of Southern California Press, 1980), 143.

11. Ross A. McFarland, "The Role of Functional versus Chronological Age Concepts in Employment of Older Workers" (Paper prepared for the Future of Retirement Policy Conference, American Institutes for Research, 29 September–1 October 1976), cited in Harold L. Sheppard and Sara E. Rix, *The Graying of Working America: The Coming Crisis in Retirement-Age Policy* (New York: Free Press, 1977), 72.

12. E.g., Stanley M. Davis, "No Connection between Executive Age and Corporate Performance," *Harvard Business Review* 57 (March–April 1979): 6.

13. E.g., Stanley R. Mohler, "Aircraft Accidents and Age," *Aging and Work* 4 (1981): 54; Davis, "No Connection."

14. E.g., Jerome A. Mark, "Measurement of Job Performance and Age," *Monthly Labor Review* 79 (December 1956): 1410; idem, "Comparative Job Performance by Age," *Monthly Labor Review* 80 (December 1957): 1470–71; Sheppard and Rix, *Graying of Working America,* 72.

15. Mark, "Comparative Job Performance" (there were changes associated with age for output per man-hour, but none for attendance); Ronald E. Kutscher and James F. Walker, "Comparative Job Performance of Office Workers by Age," *Monthly Labor Review* 83 (January 1960): 39.

16. A. T. Welford, *Ageing and Human Skill* (London: Oxford University Press, 1958), 283.

17. Ibid.

18. Fleisher and Kaplan, "Characteristics," 143.

19. Michael Fogarty, *Forty to Sixty: How We Waste the Middle Aged* (London: Center for Studies in Social Policy, 1975), 67.

20. The Secretary of Labor's report summarized the following typical studies:
    The Bureau of Business Management at the University of Illinois in a study of

supervisory ratings in manufacturing establishments in 1954 found that 11% of the workers 60 years old and over received excellent ratings for overall performance; only 3% received poor ratings. On work quality, 32% were rated better than young workers, 60% the same, and 8% poorer.

A 1959 Canadian study of salespersons in retailing showed that workers hired above the age of 40 attained higher performance ratings in a shorter period than workers hired below 30 years of age. They reached their peak performance in their fifties.

Department of Labor studies of factory production work involving physical effort indicate that a slight decrease in productivity occurs after age 45, but that the decrease does not become substantial until age 60. In office or other sedentary work, little, if any, decline occurs prior to age 60, and the subsequent decline is minor.

USDL, *The Older American Worker,* 8–9.

21. Welford, *Ageing and Human Skill,* 286.
22. Elizabeth L. Meir and Elizabeth A. Kerr, "Capabilities of Middle-Aged and Older Workers: A Survey of the Literature," *Industrial Gerontology* 3 (1976): 147, 148, citing Welford, *Ageing and Human Skill,* 283.
23. Fleisher and Kaplan, "Characteristics of Older Workers," 150.
24. *Job Re-design and Occupational Training for Older Workers* (Paris: Organization for Economic Cooperation and Development, 1965); see Doering, Rhodes, and Schuster, *The Aging Worker,* 97.
25. Stephan Griew, *Job Redesign: The Application of Biological Data on Ageing to the Design of Equipment and the Organization of Work* (Paris: Organization for Economic Cooperation and Development, 1964); G. Marbach, *Job Re-design for Older Workers: Pilot Study and Survey in Eight Member Countries* (Paris: Organization for Economic Cooperation and Development, 1968).
26. Davies and Sparrow, "Age and Work Behavior," Figs. 8.1a and 8.1b.
27. USDL, *The Older American Worker,* 9.
28. David Waldman and Bruce Avolio, "A Meta Analysis of Age Differences in Job Performance," *Journal of Applied Psychology* 71 (1986): 33–38, 37.
29. William H. Bowers, "An Appraisal of Worker Characteristics as Related to Age," *Journal of Applied Psychology* 36 (1952): 296.
30. Robert Tarnofsky, R. Ronald Shepps, and Paul J. O'Neill, "Pattern Analysis of Biographical Predictors of Success as an Insurance Salesman," *Journal of Applied Psychology* 53 (1969): 136–39.
31. Mark W. Smith, "Older Workers' Efficiency in Jobs of Various Types," *Personnel Journal* 32 (1953): 19.
32. Kutscher and Walker, "Comparative Job Performance of Office Workers by Age," 39.
33. Joseph Eisenberg, "Relationship between Age and Effects upon Work: A Study of Older Workers in the Garment Industry," *Dissertation Abstracts International* 41/04-A (1980): 1682, summarized in Doering, Rhodes, and Schuster, *The Aging Worker.*
34. U.S. Department of Labor, *Comparative Job Performance by Age: Large Plants*

in the Men's Footwear and Household Furniture Industries, Bulletin no. 1223 (Washington, D.C.: U.S. Department of Labor, 1957); see also L. Greenberg, "Productivity of Older Workers," *Gerontologist* 1 (1960): 38–41.

35. Carol H. Kelleher and Daniel A. Quirk, "Age, Functional Capacity, and Work: An Annotated Bibliography," *Industrial Gerontology* 19 (1973): 80–98.

36. Gene W. Dalton and Paul H. Thompson, "Age, Obsolescence, and Performance" (Unpublished report, 1970), cited by Davies and Sparrow, "Age and Work Behavior," 315–16; Gene W. Dalton and Paul H. Thompson, "Accelerating Obsolescence of Older Engineers," *Harvard Business Review* 49 (1971): 57–68.

37. Donald Campbell Pelz and Frank M. Andrews, *Scientists in Organizations: Productive Climates for Research and Development* (New York: John Wiley and Sons, 1966); Wayne Dennis, "Creative Productivity between the Ages of 20 and 80," in *Middle Age and Aging: A Reader in Social Psychology,* ed. Bernice L. Neugarten (Chicago: University of Chicago Press, 1968), 106.

38. Iseli Krauss, "Assessment for Retirement," in Ragan, *Work and Retirement,* 115, 117.

39. USDL, *The Older American Worker,* 9. One of the higher hiring rates for older clerical workers found during the course of the 1965 study is in the Postal Service, where appointments are made, under strict Civil Service regulations, without regard to age. Although postal clerks are engaged in some of the most physically demanding of the clerical occupations, a study made by the Bureau of Labor Statistics of the relative performance of federal mail sorters in 1963 (ibid.) showed an equal performance level for the older workers.

40. James E. Birren and K. Warner Schaie, eds., *Handbook of the Psychology of Aging* (New York: Van Nostrand Reinhold, 1977); Leonard W. Poon, ed., *Aging in the 1980s: Psychological Issues* (Washington, D.C.: American Psychological Association, 1980); Woodruff and Birren, *Aging: Scientific Perspectives and Social Issues,* 2d ed.; and Charness, *Aging and Human Performance.*

41. Doering, Rhodes, and Schuster, *The Aging Worker,* 61–82.

42. Krauss, "Assessment for Retirement," 116; K. Warner Schaie, Gisela V. Labouvie, and Barbara U. Buech, "Generational and Cohort-Specific Differences in Adult Cognitive Functioning: A Fourteen-Year Study of Independent Samples," *Developmental Psychology* 9 (1973): 151; Jack Botwinick, "Intellectual Abilities," in Birren and Schaie, *Handbook of the Psychology of Aging,* 580.

43. K. Warner Schaie, "Age Changes in Adult Intelligence," in Woodruff and Birren, *Aging: Scientific Perspectives and Social Issues.*

44. See, e.g., Joseph D. Matorazzo, *Wechsler's Measurement and Appraisal of Adult Intelligence,* 5th ed. (Baltimore: Williams and Wilkins, 1972), 226, table 9.5.

45. Nancy A. Newton, Lawrence W. Lazarus, and Jack Weinberg, "Aging: Biopsychosocial Perspectives," in *Normality and the Life Cycle: A Critical Integration,* ed. Daniel Offer and Melvin Sabshin (New York: Basic Books, 1984), 262–66.

46. Schaie, "Adult Intelligence," 143.

47. Ibid., 145.

48. Ibid.

49. Letter from James E. Birren, 6 January 1986.
50. Schaie, "Adult Intelligence," 145.
51. Ibid., 146; see also Schaie, Labouvie, and Buech, "Cognitive Functioning."
52. John L. Horn and Raymond B. Cattell, "Age Differences in Fluid and Crystallized Intelligence," *Acta Psychologica* 26 (1967): 107; Schaie, Labouvie, and Buech, "Cognitive Functioning."
53. James E. Birren, Walter R. Cunningham, and Koichi Yamamoto, "Psychology of Adult Development and Aging," *Annual Review of Psychology* 34 (1983): 549.
54. Ibid., 550, summarizing Schaie et al.
55. Ibid., 551–52.
56. Davies and Sparrow, "Age and Work Behavior." The literature is reviewed by John F. Corso, "Auditory Perception and Communication," in Birren and Schaie, *Handbook of the Psychology of Aging;* D. R. Davies, "Age Differences in Paced Inspection Tasks," in *Human Aging and Behavior: Recent Advances in Research and Theory,* ed. George A. Talland (New York: Academic Press, 1968); D. R. Davies, D. M. Jones, and Ann Taylor, "Selective and Sustained Attention Tasks: Individual and Group Differences," in *Varieties of Attention,* ed. Raja Parasuraman and D. R. Davies (New York: Academic Press, 1984); Donald H. Kausler, "Episodic Memory: Memorizing Performance," in Charness, *Aging and Human Performance;* Dana J. Plude and William J. Hoyer, "Attention and Performance: Identifying and Localizing Age Deficits," ibid.; A. T. Welford, "Motor Performance," in Birren and Schaie, *Handbook of the Psychology of Aging.*
57. James E. Birren and M. Virtrue Williams, "Speed of Behavior," in Poon, *Aging in the 1980s;* Welford, "Motor Performance," 450.
58. Welford, "Motor Performance"; Barry Layton, "Perceptual Noise and Aging," *Psychological Bulletin* 82 (1975): 875; Corso, "Auditory Perception and Communication"; James L. Fozard, Ernst Wolf, Benjamin Bell, Ross A. McFarland, and Stephen Podolsky, "Visual Perception and Communication," in Birren and Schaie, *Handbook of the Psychology of Aging.*
59. D. R. Davies and S. Griew, "Age and Vigilance" in *Behavior, Aging, and the Nervous System,* ed. A. T. Welford and J. E. Birren (Springfield, Ill.: Charles C. Thomas, 1965); D. R. Davies and Raja Parasuraman, *The Psychology of Vigilance* (London: Academic Press, 1982).
60. F. Hywel Murrell, "The Effects of Extensive Practice on Age Differences in Reaction Time," *Journal of Gerontology* 25 (1970): 268–74.
61. K. F. H. Murrell, P. F. Powesland, and Bel Forsaith, "A Study of Pillar-Driving in Relation to Age," *Occupational Psychology* 3 (1962): 45–52.
62. David A. Walsh, "Age Differences in Learning and Memory," in Woodruff and Birren, *Aging: Scientific Perspectives and Social Issues,* 165.
63. Ibid., 172, 174 (quotation).
64. James L. Fozard, "The Time for Remembering," in Poon, *Aging in the 1980s,* 273.
65. David A. Walsh and Mariette Baldwin, "Age Differences in Integrated Semantic Memory," *Developmental Psychology* 13 (1977): 509–14; Kathryn J. Waddell

and Barbara Rogoff, "Effect of Contextual Organization on Spatial Memory of Middle-Aged and Older Women," *Developmental Psychology* 17 (1981): 878–85.

66. Birren, Cunningham, and Yamamoto, "Adult Development and Aging," 555.
67. Walsh, "Age Differences in Learning and Memory," 173.
68. See Newton, Lazarus, and Weinberg, "Aging: Biopsychosocial Perspectives."
69. J. A. Stern, P. J. Oster, and K. Newport, "Reaction Time Measures, Hemisphere Specialization, and Age," in Poon, *Aging in the 1980s*, 309.
70. James E. Birren, Anita M. Woods, and M. Virtrue Williams, "Behavioral Slowing with Age: Causes, Organization, and Consequences," in Poon, *Aging in the 1980s*, 302.
71. Ibid.
72. Newton, Lazarus, and Weinberg, "Aging: Biopsychosocial Perspectives."
73. Birren, Cunningham, and Yamamoto, "Adult Development and Aging," 552.
74. Horn and Cattell, "Fluid and Crystallized Intelligence." See also John L. Horn and Raymond B. Cattell, "Age Differences in Primary Mental Ability Factors," *Journal of Gerontology* 21 (1966): 210–20; Paul B. Baltes and K. Warner Schaie, "Aging and IQ: The Myth of the Twilight Years," *Psychology Today* 7 (March 1974): 35; Botwinick, "Intellectual Abilities."
75. The debate includes Horn and Cattell's 1966 and 1967 proposal, Schaie's statement of his position as of 1974, the criticism of it by Horn and Donaldson in 1976, and the Baltes and Schaie restatement of their position in 1976. The debate is summarized in Robert Sternberg and Cynthia Berg, "What Are Theories of Adult Intellectual Development Theories Of?" in *Cognitive Functioning and Social Structure Over the Life Course*, ed. Carmi Schooler and K. Warner Schaie (Norwood, N.J.: Ablex, 1987), 1–23.
76. K. Warner Schaie and Kathy Gribben, "Adult Development and Aging," *Annual Review of Psychology* 26 (1975): 65, emphasizing the findings of Schaie, Labouvie, and Buech, "Cognitive Functioning," 151, and K. Warner Schaie and Gisela Labouvie-Vief, "Generational Versus Ontogenetic Components of Change in Adult Cognitive Behavior: A Fourteen-Year Cross-Sequential Study," *Developmental Psychology* 10 (1974): 305; see also Baltes and Schaie, "Aging and IQ." These conclusions have been criticized; see, e.g., John L. Horn and Gary Donaldson, "On the Myth of Intellectual Decline," *American Psychologist* 31 (1976): 701. See generally Birren, Cunningham, and Yamamoto, "Adult Development and Aging," 548–49.
77. Doering, Rhodes, and Schuster, *The Aging Worker*, 61.
78. Ibid., 63.
79. Ibid., 196.
80. Dan Baugher, "Is the Older Worker Inherently Incompetent?" *Aging and Work* 1 (1978): 248.
81. Jack Botwinick, "Intellectual Abilities," in Birren and Schaie, *Handbook of the Psychology of Aging*. See also Jack Botwinick, *Aging and Behavior* (New York: Springer, 1984), ch. 14.
82. Botwinick, "Intellectual Abilities," 590.

Chapter 14. Individualized Determination of Productivity

1. *Forms of Wage and Salary Payment for High Productivity* (Paris: Organization for Economic Cooperation and Development, 1970), cited in H. Suzuki, "Age, Seniority, and Wages," *International Labour Review* 113 (1976): 73–74 (measurement difficulties involved in payment by results).
2. James J. Healy, "The Ability Factor in Labor Relations," *Arbitration Journal* 10 (1955): 10, cited in Suzuki, "Age, Seniority, and Wages," 71.
3. Vance v. Bradley, 440 U.S. 93, 103, n. 20 (1979).
4. Irwin Ross, "Retirement at Seventy: A New Trauma for Management," *Fortune*, 8 May 1978, 110.
5. Jeffrey Sonnenfeld, "Dealing with the Aging Work Force," *Harvard Business Review* 56 (November—December 1978): 81.
6. Iseli Krauss, "Assessment for Retirement," in *Work and Retirement: Policy Issues,* ed. Pauline K. Ragan (Los Angeles: University of Southern California Press, 1980), 121; Lee J. Cronbach, "New Light on Test Strategy from Decision Theory" (Paper presented at Invitational Conference on Testing Problems, Educational Testing Service, Princeton, N.J., 1954), reprinted in *Testing Problems in Perspective,* ed. Anne Anastasi (Washington, D.C.: American Council on Education, 1966).
7. Krauss, "Assessment," 122.
8. Adam Bruce Rowland, "Age Discrimination in Retirement: In Search of an Alternative," *American Journal of Law and Medicine* 8 (1983): 449.
9. EEOC v. Pennsylvania, 596 F. Supp. 1333, 1341 (D. Pa. 1984); see also EEOC v. Los Angeles County, 706 F.2d 1039, 1043 (9th Cir. 1983).
10. Vandra L. Huber, "An Analysis of Performance Appraisal Practices in the Public Sector: A Review and Recommendation," *Public Personnel Management* 12 (Fall 1983): 258; Charles M. Kelly, "Reasonable Performance Appraisals," *Training and Development Journal* 38 (January 1984): 79.
11. Mildred Doering, Susan R. Rhodes, and Michael Schuster, *The Aging Worker: Research and Recommendations* (Beverly Hills: Sage, 1983), 89–104.
12. The term is an acronym for *G*eneral Physique, *U*pper Extremities, *L*ower Extremities, *H*earing, *E*yesight, *M*entality, and *P*ersonality. Leon Koyl, *Employing the Older Worker: Matching the Employee to the Job,* 2d ed. (Washington, D.C.: National Council on Aging, 1974), 32. Developed by Koyl, a Canadian medical consultant, the test was popularized in the United States by the National Council on Aging. See generally Michael D. Batten, "Application of a Unique Industrial Health System," *Industrial Gerontology* 19 (1973): 38; Mary Youry, "GULHEMP: What Workers *Can* Do," *Manpower* 7 (June 1975): 4.
13. Gerald Maguire of Bankers Life and Casualty, quoted in Henry M. Wallfesh, *The Effects of Extending the Mandatory Retirement Age* (New York: AMACOM, A Division of American Management Assoc., 1978), 36–37.
14. Donnelly v. Exxon Research and Engineering Co., 12 Fair Empl. Cas. (BNA) 417 (D.N.J. 1974), *aff'd mem.,* 521 F.2d 1398 (3d Cir. 1975), concerned a

performance-based plan in which the least-productive employees were laid off for financial reasons. The plan, which included termination for "technological obsolescence" (ibid. at 420), was approved by the court.

15. *"Here again, the strongest indication of the lack of real basis for most age limitations is the demonstrated willingness of so many American employers to consider older workers on their merits as individuals and to hire them.* Although one out of every five of the employers included in the 1965 Employment Service survey hired no new employees among applicants over 45 years of age, another one-fifth hired at least 15 percent in this age group. Many of these firms reported an active policy of recruiting older persons, and praised them for performance and dependability." U.S. Department of Labor, *The Older American Worker: Age Discrimination in Employment, Report of Secretary of Labor to Congress under Section 715 of Civil Rights Act of 1964* (Washington, D.C.: U.S. Government Printing Office, 1965), 9.

16. See also, e.g., Harland Fox, "Utilization of Older Manpower," *Harvard Business Review* 29 (November 1951): 40.

17. Clifford M. Baumbeck, *Structural Wage Issues in Collective Bargaining* (Lexington, Mass.: Heath, 1971), 44–45, cited in Suzuki, "Age, Seniority, and Wages," 74.

18. David Waldman and Bruce Avolio, "A Meta Analysis of Age Difference in Job Performance," *Journal of Applied Psychology* 71 (1986): 37.

19. George W. Torrence, "Salary Reviews and Performance Appraisals," *Conference Board Record* (February 1964): 46–47.

20. U.S. Department of Labor, *Interim Report to Congress on Age Discrimination in Employment Act Studies, Report to the Congress Required by Section 5 of the Age Discrimination in Employment Act,* prepared for the U.S. Congress by Malcolm H. Morrison and Betty H. Roberts (Washington, D.C.: U.S. Government Printing Office, 1982) 85, table 20.

21. Western Airlines v. Criswell, 472 U.S. 400 (1985).

22. 23 September 1986, *Congressional Record,* 99th Cong., 2d sess., 132: H8132–38 (statements of Reps. Murphy, Rinaldo, Roukema, and Hughes).

Chapter 15. Attitudes toward the Elderly

1. See generally Jack Levin and William C. Levin, *Ageism: Prejudice and Discrimination against the Elderly* (Belmont, Calif.: Wadsworth, 1980).

2. Address by U.S. Representative Claude Pepper, in *Final Report of the 1981 White House Conference on Aging* (Washington, D.C.: U.S. Government Printing Office, 1981), 2:48.

3. Robert N. Butler, *Why Survive? Being Old in America* (New York: Harper and Row, 1975), 6. See also Chapter 17, below.

4. E.g., Ruth Bennett and Judith Eckman, "Attitudes toward Aging: A Critical Examination of Recent Literature and Implications for Future Research," in *The Psychology of Adult Development and Aging,* ed. Carl Eisdorfer and M. Powell

Lawton (Washington, D.C.: American Psychological Association, 1973). This section draws heavily on Neil S. Lutsky, "Attitudes toward Old Age and Elderly Persons," *Annual Review of Gerontology and Geriatrics* 1 (1980): 287.

5. Donald G. McTavish, "Perceptions of Old People: A Review of Research Methodologies and Findings," *Gerontologist* 11 (1971): 90.

6. Bennett and Eckman, "Attitudes," 592.

7. E.g., Robert C. Atchley, *The Social Forces in Later Life: An Introduction to Social Gerontology,* 2d ed. (Belmont, Calif.: Wadsworth, 1977); Butler, *Why Survive?;* Russell A. Ward, "The Impact of Subjective Age and Stigma on Older Persons," *Journal of Gerontology* 32 (1977): 227.

8. See Atchley, *Social Forces in Later Life;* Vern L. Bengston, *The Social Psychology of Aging,* (Indianapolis: Bobbs-Merrill, 1973); Butler, *Why Survive?;* Louis Harris and Associates, Inc., *The Myth and Reality of Aging in America* (Washington, D.C.: National Council on the Aging, 1975); William Graham Sumner, *Folkways* (Boston: Ginn, 1907); Staff of House Select Committee on Aging, *Mandatory Retirement: The Social and Human Costs of Enforced Idleness,* 95th Cong., 1st sess., 1977, Committee Print; Robert N. Butler, "Ageism: Another Form of Bigotry," *Gerontologist* 9 (1969): 243; Leland J. Davies, "Attitudes toward Old Age and Aging as Shown by Humor," *Gerontologist* 17 (1977): 220; George L. Maddox, "Growing Old: Getting beyond the Stereotypes," in *Foundations of Practical Gerontology,* ed. Rosamonde Ramsay Boyd and Charles G. Oakes (Columbia: University of South Carolina Press, 1969); Erdman B. Palmore, "Social and Economic Aspects of Aging," in *Geriatric Psychiatry: A Handbook for Psychiatrists and Primary-Care Physicians,* ed. Leopold Bellak, Toksoz Karasu, and Caroline Birenbaum (New York: Grune and Stratton, 1976); idem, "Facts on Aging: A Short Quiz," *Gerontologist* 17 (1977): 315; idem, "Advantages of Aging," *Gerontologist* 19 (1979): 221; Erdman B. Palmore and Kenneth Manton, "Ageism Compared to Racism and Sexism," *Journal of Gerontology* 28 (1973): 363; Erdman B. Palmore and Frank Whittington, "Trends in the Relative Status of the Aged," *Social Forces* 50 (1971): 84; Rosalie H. Rosenfeld, "The Elderly Mystique," *Journal of Social Issues* 21 (October 1965): 37; Timothy Weber and Paul Cameron, "Comment: Humor and Aging—A Response," *Gerontologist* 18 (1978): 73.

9. Butler, *Why Survive?* 6–16.

10. Louis Harris and Associates, *Myth and Reality.*

11. Levin and Levin, *Ageism,* 85.

12. Joseph M. Holtzman and Hiroko Akiyama, "What Children See: The Aged on Television in Japan and the United States," *Gerontologist* 25 (1985): 62; Robert W. Kubey, "Television and Aging: Past, Present, and Future," *Gerontologist* 20 (1980): 16; Craig Aronoff, "Old Age in Prime Time," *Journal of Communication* 24 (Autumn 1974): 86; James M. Bishop and Daniel R. Krause, "Depictions of Aging and Old Age on Saturday Morning Television," *Gerontologist* 24 (1984): 91; Herbert C. Northcott, "Too Young, Too Old—Age in the World of Television," *Gerontologist* 15 (1975): 184; Nancy Signorielli and George Gerbner, "The Image of the Elderly in Prime-Time Television Drama," *Generations* 3 (Fall 1978): 10.

13. Lutsky, "Attitudes toward Old Age."
14. U.S. Department of Labor, *The Older American Worker: Age Discrimination in Employment, Report of Secretary of Labor to Congress under Section 715 of Civil Rights Act of 1964* (Washington, D.C.: U.S. Government Printing Office, 1965), 5–6.
15. Ibid., 2.
16. *Congressional Record,* 1967, 113: 34742 (statement of Rep. Burke).
17. Palmore, "Advantages of Aging." For example, the elderly have better governmental support than most of the poor, and they occupy a greater percentage of public housing than their numbers alone would suggest. Elizabeth A. Kutzka, "Toward an Aging Policy," *Social Policy* 12 (May–June 1981): 39. See also Samuel H. Preston, "Children and the Elderly in the U.S.," *Scientific American* 251 (December 1984): 44.
18. E. Jones, "The Significance of the Grandfather for the Fate of the Individual," *Internationale Zeitschrift für Ärztliche Pschoanalyze* 1 (1913): 210, reprinted in *Papers on Psychoanalysis,* 4th ed. (New Haven: Yale University Press, 1938).
19. Mildred Doering, Susan R. Rhodes, and Michael Schuster, *The Aging Worker: Research and Recommendations* (Beverly Hills: Sage, 1983), 61; see also ibid., table C-1, Appendix.
20. James E. Haefner, "Race, Age, Sex, and Competence as Factors in Employer Selection of the Disadvantaged," *Journal of Applied Psychology* 62 (1977): 199; Jean O. Britton and Kenneth R. Thomas, "Age and Sex as Employment Variables: Views of Employment Service Interviewers," *Journal of Employment Counseling* 10 (1973): 180; James A. Craft, Samuel I. Doctors, Yitzchak M. Skhop, and Thomas J. Benecki, "Simulated Management Perceptions, Hiring Decisions, and Age," *Aging and Work* 2 (1979): 95; Benson Rosen and Thomas H. Jerdee, "The Influence of Age Stereotypes on Managerial Decisions," *Journal of Applied Psychology* 61 (1976): 428; idem, "The Nature of Job-Related Age Stereotypes," ibid., 180.
21. Jacob Tuckman and Irving Lorge, "Attitudes toward Old Workers," *Journal of Applied Psychology* 36 (1952): 149.
22. Rosen and Jerdee, "The Nature of Job-Related Age Stereotypes."
23. Rosen and Jerdee, "The Influence of Age Stereotypes on Managerial Decisions," 431.
24. Benson Rosen and Thomas H. Jerdee, "Too Old or Not Too Old," *Harvard Business Review* 55 (November–December 1977): 97.
25. Britton and Thomas, "Employment Variables."
26. Ibid.
27. Louis Harris and Associates, *Myth and Reality.*
28. "Finds Employers Favor No Age Bar," *New York Times,* 21 March 1929, 23.
29. Dwight L. Palmer and John A. Brownell, "Influence of Age on Employment Opportunities," *Monthly Labor Review* 48 (April 1939): 778.
30. Ibid.
31. Vern L. Bengtson, Patricia L. Kasschau, and Pauline K. Ragan, "The Impact of Social Structure on Aging Individuals," in *The Handbook of the Psychology of Aging,* ed. James E. Birren and K. Warner Schaie (New York: Van Nostrand Reinhold, 1977), 327.

32. Lutsky, "Attitudes toward Old Age," 289.
33. E.g., Timothy H. Brubaker and Edward A. Powers, "The Stereotype of 'Old': A Review and Alternative Approach," *Journal of Gerontology* 31 (1976): 441; Kogan, "Beliefs, Attitudes, and Stereotypes about Old People: A New Look at Some Old Issues," *Research on Aging* 1 (1979).
34. Lutsky, "Attitudes toward Old Age," 290. See, e.g., Bengtson, Kasschau, and Ragan, "The Impact of Social Structure on Aging Individuals"; Butler, *Why Survive?* 6–7; Ethel Shanas, "Social Myth as Hypothesis: The Case of the Family Relations of Old People," *Gerontologist* 19 (1979): 3; Clark Tibbitts, "Can We Invalidate Negative Stereotypes of Aging?" *Gerontologist* 19 (1979): 10.
35. Lutsky, "Attitudes toward Old Age," 313.
36. Ibid., 327.

Chapter 16. Stereotypes and Cognitive Error

1. E.g., Daniel Kahneman, Paul Slovic, and Amos Tversky, *Judgment under Uncertainty: Heuristics and Biases* (New York: Cambridge University Press, 1982); Sarah Lichtenstein and Baruch Fischoff, "Do Those Who Know More Also Know More about How Much They Know?" *Organizational Behavior and Human Performance* 20 (1977): 159–83; Richard Nisbett and Lee Ross, *Human Inference: Strategies and Shortcomings of Social Judgement* (Englewood Cliffs, N.J.: Prentice-Hall, 1980); Ward Edwards and Detlof von Winterfeldt, "Cognitive Illusions and Their Implications for the Law," *Southern California Law Review* 59 (1986): 225; Robin M. Hogarth, *Judgment and Choice: The Psychology of Decisions* (New York: Wiley, 1980).
2. See note 1.
3. Also see Clark McCauley, Christopher L. Still, and Mary Segal, "Stereotyping: From Prejudice to Prediction," *Psychological Bulletin* 87 (1980): 195.
4. For example, a heading "What Is the Motive Behind Stereotypes?" is followed immediately by the sentence, "First, what exactly is the motive for prejudice?" Nisbett and Ross, *Human Inference,* 237.
5. Ibid., 238.
6. Ibid., 239.
7. Ibid., 241.
8. Daniel Kahneman and Amos Tversky, "Subjective Probability: A Judgment of Representativeness," *Cognitive Psychology* 3 (1972): 430; Kahneman and Tversky, "On the Psychology of Prediction," *Psychological Review* 80 (1973): 237.

Chapter 17. Prejudice, Ambivalence, and Psychoanalysis

1. Sigmund Freud, "Totem and Taboo" (1913–14), in *The Standard Edition of the Complete Psychological Works of Sigmund Freud,* ed. and trans. James Strachey

(London: Hogarth Press and the Institute of Psychoanalysis, 1975), vol. 13; P. Radford, "Ambivalence," in *Basic Psychoanalytic Concepts of Metapsychology, Conflicts, Anxiety, and Other Subjects,* ed. Humberto Najera (New York: Basic Books, 1970).

2. Juanita Kreps, "Employment Policy and Income Maintenance for the Aged," in *Aging and Social Policy,* ed. John C. McKinney and Frank T. Devyver (New York: Appleton-Century-Crofts, 1966).

3. David Schwiebert, "Unfavorable Stereotyping of the Aged as a Function of Death Anxiety, Sex, Perception of Elderly Relatives, and a Death Anxiety-Repression" (Ph.D. diss., Auburn University, 1978).

4. Sigmund Freud, "The Dynamics of Transference," *Standard Edition,* vol. 12.

5. Margaret Blenkner, "Social Work and Family Relationships in Later Life, with Some Thoughts on Filial Maturity," in *Social Structure and the Family: Generational Relations,* ed. Ethel Shanas and Gordon F. Streib (Englewood Cliffs, N.J.: Prentice-Hall, 1965); Robert N. Butler, *Why Survive? Being Old in America* (New York: Harper and Row, 1975); Freud, "Totem and Taboo"; Irving Sternschein, "The Experience of Separation-Individual in Infancy and Its Reverberations through the Course of Life: Maturity, Senescence, and Sociological Implications," *Journal of the American Psychoanalytic Association* 21 (1973): 633–45.

6. On avoidance of the aged, Richard A. Kalish, "Social Distance and the Dying," *Community Mental Health Journal* 2 (1966): 152; W. W. Meissner, "Affective Response to Psychoanalytic Death Symbols," *Journal of Abnormal and Social Psychology* 56 (1958): 295; Phyllis Mutschler, "Factors Affecting Choice of and Perseveration in Social Work with the Aged," *Gerontologist* 11 (1971): 231; John J. Spinetta, David Rigler, and Myron Karon, "Personal Space as a Measure of a Dying Child's Sense of Isolation," *Journal of Consulting and Clinical Psychology* 42 (1974): 751. See also Herman Feifel, "Attitudes toward Death: A Psychological Perspective," *Journal of Consulting and Clinical Psychology* 33 (1969): 292.

7. Charles A. Salter and Carlota de Lerma Salter, "Attitudes toward Aging and Behaviors toward the Elderly among Young People as a Function of Death Anxiety," *Gerontologist* 16 (1976): 232.

8. James A. Thorson and Spenser Ackerman, "Attitudes toward the Aged and Frequency of Thoughts about Death," *Psychological Reports* 37 (1975): 825–26, cited in Schwiebert, "Unfavorable Stereotyping." See also Robert Kastenbaum, "Death, Dying, and Bereavement in Old Age: New Developments and Their Possible Implications for Psychosocial Care," *Aged Care and Services Review* 1 (May–June 1978): 1.

9. Ernest Becker, *The Denial of Death* (New York: Free Press, 1973).

10. Schwiebert, "Unfavorable Stereotyping."

11. Cf. Jaber F. Gubrium, *The Myth of the Golden Years: A Socioeconomic Theory of Aging* (Springfield, Ill.: Thomas, 1973).

12. Manfred F. R. Kets de Vries, ed., *The Irrational Executive: Psychoanalytic Studies in Management* (New York: International University Press, 1984), xvi.

13. Herbert A. Simon, *Administrative Behavior: A Study of Decision-Making Processes in Administrative Organization* (New York: Free Press, 1976).

14. Douglas LaBier, "Irrational Behavior in Bureaucracy," in Kets de Vries, *The Irrational Executive*.

15. Joel Kovel, "Rationalization and the Family," in *Capitalism and Infancy: Essays on Psychoanalysis and Politics,* ed. Barry Richards (Atlantic Highlands, N.J.: Humanities Press, 1984), 117.

16. Harry Levinson, *Emotional Health in the World of Work* (New York: Harper and Row, 1964), ch. 18.

17. Isabel E. P. Menzies, "A Case-Study in the Functioning of Social Systems as a Defense against Anxiety: A Report on a Study of the Nursing Service of a General Hospital," *Human Relations* 13 (1960): 95.

18. Bernard Diamond, "The Children of Leviathan: Psychoanalytic Speculations Concerning Welfare Law and Punitive Sanctions," *California Law Review* 54 (1966): 364.

19. Joe R. Feagin, *Subordinating the Poor: Welfare and American Beliefs* (Englewood Cliffs, N.J.: Prentice-Hall, 1975).

20. Charles R. Lawrence III, "The Id, The Ego, and Equal Protection: Reckoning with Unconscious Racism," *Stanford Law Review* 39 (1987): 322.

21. Ibid.

22. Ibid., 322, n. 22. See Personnel Administrator v. Feeney, 442 U.S. 256 (1979); Marjorie J. Weinzweig, "Discriminatory Impact and Intent under the Equal Protection Clause: The Supreme Court and the Mind-Body Problem," *Law and Inequality* 1 (1983): 277.

23. Lawrence, "The Id," 322, n. 22. See, e.g., Richard A. Wasserstrom, "Racism, Sexism, and Preferential Treatment: An Approach to the Topics," *UCLA Law Review* 24 (1977): 581, 590.

24. Lawrence, "The Id," 317.

25. Herbert Hendin, Willard Gaylin, and Arthur Carr, *Psychoanalysis and Social Research: The Psychoanalytic Study of the Non-Patient* (Garden City, N.Y.: Doubleday, 1965).

26. Leland J. Davies, "Attitudes toward Old Age and Aging as Shown by Humor," *Gerontologist* 17 (1977): 220; Erdman Palmore, "Attitudes toward Aging as Shown by Humor," *Gerontologist* 11 (1971): 181; Timothy Weber and Paul Cameron, "Comment: Humor and Aging—A Response," *Gerontologist* 18 (1978): 73.

27. Juanita Kreps, "A Case Study of Variables in Retirement Policy," *Monthly Labor Review* 84 (June 1961): 587; U.S. Department of Labor, *The Older American Worker: Age Discrimination in Employment, Report of Secretary of Labor to Congress under Section 715 of Civil Rights Act of 1964, Research Materials* (Washington, D.C.: U.S. Government Printing Office, 1965).

28. David T. Barker and Robert L. Clark, "Mandatory Retirement and Labor-Force Participation of Respondents in the Retirement History Study," *Social Security Bulletin* 43 (November 1980): 20–29.

29. Wayne K. Kirchner and Marvin D. Dunnette, "Survey of Union Policy toward

Older Workers," *Journal of Personnel, Administration, and Industrial Relations* 1 (1954): 156.

30. George Mandler, *Mind and Emotion* (Melbourne, Fl.: Krieger, 1975).

31. Richard Nisbett and Lee Ross, *Human Inference: Strategies and Shortcomings of Social Judgment* (Englewood Cliffs, N.J.: Prentice-Hall, 1980), 242.

32. Ibid., 243.

33. Ibid., 245.

34. Cf. Michael S. Moore, *Law and Psychiatry: Rethinking the Relationship* (New York: Cambridge University Press, 1984).

35. Personal communication with the late Miss Anna Freud, 7 June 1980.

36. Richard M. Cohn, "Contract and Discrimination in Retirement Policy: An Evaluation of Lazear's 'Mandatory Retirement' " (n.p., 1981); Lester C. Thurow, *Generating Inequality: Mechanisms of Distribution in the U.S. Economy* (New York: Basic Books, 1975); Richard A. Posner, *The Economics of Justice* (Cambridge: Harvard University Press, 1981).

37. Gary S. Becker, *The Economics of Discrimination*, 2d ed. (Chicago: University of Chicago Press, 1971).

38. Nisbett and Ross, *Human Inference*, 237–42.

39. E.g., J. Morris Clark, "Legislative Motivation and Fundamental Rights in Constitutional Law," *San Diego Law Review* 15 (1978): 954; Larry Simon, "Racially Prejudiced Governmental Actions: A Motivation Theory of the Constitutional Ban against Racial Discrimination," *San Diego Law Review* 15 (1978): 1041.

40. Griffin v. Breckenridge, 403 U.S. 99 (1971). The statute was 42 U.S.C., § 1985(3) (1982).

41. Palmer v. Thompson, 403 U.S. 217, 224–26 (1971).

42. Washington v. Davis, 426 U.S. 229, 238–48 (1976); see also Hunter v. Underwood, 471 U.S. 222 (1985), citing Village of Arlington Heights v. Metropolitan Housing Development Corp., 429 U.S. 252, 264–65 (1977), following Washington v. Davis, 426 U.S. 229 (1976). See generally "Colloquium on Legislative and Administrative Motivation in Constitutional Law," *San Diego Law Review* 15 (1978): 925; Paul Brest, "Palmer v. Thompson: An Approach to the Problem of Unconstitutional Legislative Motive," *Supreme Court Review* 1971, 95; John H. Ely, "Legislative and Administrative Motivation in Constitutional Law," *Yale Law Journal* 79 (1970): 1205.

43. United States v. Carolene Products Co., 304 U.S. 144, 152 n. 4.

Chapter 18.   The Psychology of the Work Place

1. D. L. Leslie, *The Economics of Labor Law: Unions and Bargaining Units* (Working Paper No. 12, Stanford Law School Law & Economics Program, Working Paper Series, 1983).

2. G. Boglietti, "Discrimination against Older Workers and the Promotion of Equality and Opportunity," *International Labour Review* 110 (1974): 355.

3. Harry Levinson, *Emotional Health in the World of Work* (New York: Harper and Row, 1964), ch. 18.

4. Lawrence M. Friedman, *Your Time Will Come: The Law of Age Discrimination and Mandatory Retirement* (New York: Russell Sage Foundation, 1984).

5. Harrison Givens, Jr., "An Evaluation of Mandatory Retirement," *Annals of the American Academy of Political and Social Science* 438 (1978): 51.

6. Max Weber, *Economy and Society,* ed. Guenther Roth and Claus Wittich (New York: Bedminster Press, 1968), 2: 656–57.

7. Henry S. Farber and Daniel H. Saks, "Why Workers Want Unions: The Role of Relative Wages and Job Characteristics," *Journal of Political Economy* 88 (1980): 349.

8. Oliver E. Williamson, *Markets and Hierarchies, Analysis and Antitrust Implications: A Study in the Economics of Internal Organization* (New York: Free Press, 1975), 75.

9. Jack S. Futterman, "Administrative Developments in the Social Security Program since 1965," *Social Security Bulletin* 35 (April 1972): 6.

10. Williamson, *Markets and Hierarchies,* 75.

11. Charles M. Kelly, "Reasonable Performance Appraisals," *Training and Development Journal* 38 (January 1984): 79.

12. Juanita M. Kreps, "A Case Study of Variables in Retirement Policy," *Monthly Labor Review* 84 (June 1961): 587.

13. Clarence D. Long, *The Labor Force under Changing Income and Employment,* National Bureau of Economic Research, General series no. 65 (Princeton: Princeton University Press, 1958), 168, n. 31.

14. Kreps, "Case Study of Variables"; Beatrice Brower, *Retirement of Employees: Policies, Procedures, Practices,* Studies in Personnel Policy, no. 148 (New York: National Industrial Conference Board, 1955); Margaret S. Gordon, "The Older Worker and Retirement Policies," *Monthly Labor Review* 83 (June 1960): 577.

15. U.S. Department of Labor, Bureau of Employment Security, *Counseling and Placement Services for Older Workers,* BES no. E152 (Washington, D.C.: U.S. Government Printing Office, 1956), summarized in Abraham Stahler, "Job Problems and Their Solutions," *Monthly Labor Review* 80 (January 1957): 22.

16. Joseph J. Spengler, "The Aged and Public Policy," in *Behavior and Adaptation in Late Life,* ed. Ewald W. Busse and Eric Pfeiffer (Boston: Little, Brown, 1969), 382.

17. David T. Barker and Robert L. Clark, "Mandatory Retirement and Labor-Force Participation of Respondents in the Retirement History Study," *Social Security Bulletin* 43 (November 1980): 20–29.

18. "Causes of Discrimination against Older Workers," *Monthly Labor Review* 46 (May 1938): 1139.

19. E.g., K. Bers, *Union Policy and the Older Worker* (Berkeley, Calif.: Institute of Industrial Relations, 1957).

20. Morton Deutsch, *Distributive Justice: A Social-Psychological Perspective* (New Haven: Yale University Press, 1985).

Chapter 19.   The Four Models

1. Robert M. MacDonald, *Mandatory Retirement and the Law* (Washington, D.C.: American Enterprise for Public Policy Research, 1978).
2. The form of the argument here is drawn from Morley Gunderson and James E. Pesando, "Eliminating Mandatory Retirement: Economics and Human Rights," *Canadian Public Policy—Analyse de Politiques* 6 (1982): 352; see also MacDonald, *Mandatory Retirement and the Law.*
3. Eugene Emerson Jennings, *Routes to the Executive Suite* (New York: McGraw-Hill, 1951).
4. U.S. Department of Labor, *Interim Report to Congress on Age Discrimination in Employment Act Studies, Report to the Congress Required by Section 5 of the Age Discrimination in Employment Act,* prepared for the U.S. Congress by Malcolm H. Morrison and Betty H. Roberts (Washington, D.C.: U.S. Government Printing Office, 1982), 62.
5. David T. Barker and Robert L. Clark, "Mandatory Retirement and Labor-Force Participation in the Retirement History Study," *Social Security Bulletin* 43 (November 1980): 29.
6. Daniel Seligman, "Keeping Up: The Case for Ageism," *Fortune,* 20 September 1982, 47.
7. Richard Cohn, "Quantitative Evidence of Age Discrimination: Some Theoretical Issues and Their Consequences," *Aging and Work* 3 (1980): 149.
8. U.S. Department of Labor, *The Older American Worker: Age Discrimination in Employment, Report of Secretary of Labor to Congress under Section 715 of Civil Rights Act of 1964* (Washington, D.C.: U.S. Government Printing Office, 1965), 12; Milton L. Barron, *The Aging American* (Westport, Conn.: Greenwood, 1974), 40.
9. "Finds Employers Favor No Age Bar," *New York Times,* 21 March 1929, 23.
10. USDL, *The Older American Worker: Research Materials.*
11. Western Airlines v. Criswell, 472 U.S. 400 (1985); Usery v. Tamiami Trail Tours, Inc., 532 F.2d 224 (5th Cir. 1975).
12. Personal communications, Frances Raday.
13. See generally Frederic M. Scherer, *Industrial Market Structure and Economic Performance,* 2d ed. (Boston: Houghton Mifflin, 1980), 345–47.
14. Jerry M. Flint, "Businesses Fear Major Problems from Later Age of Retirement," *New York Times,* 2 October 1977, 1.
15. Ibid., 1.
16. Barker and Clark, "Mandatory Retirement."
17. Galenson quoted by Flint, "Businesses Fear Major Problems," 38. Looking at the converse situation, a 1982 study found that affirmative action employment programs favoring women and members of minority groups do not have a negative effect on the treatment of older workers. Usually, there is no effect; occasionally, treatment of older workers is improved by affirmative action. Benson

Rosen, Thomas H. Jerdee, and John Huonker, "Are Older Workers Hurt by Affirmative Action?" *Business Horizons* 25 (September–October 1982): 67.

18. Massachusetts Board of Retirement v. Murgia, 427 U.S. 307, 314–15 (1976); Wilma Donahue, Harold L. Orbach, and Otto Pollak, "Retirement: The Emerging Social Pattern," in *Handbook of Social Gerontology: Societal Aspects of Aging,* ed. Clark Tibbitts (Chicago: University of Chicago Press, 1960).

19. Lawrence Tribe, *American Constitutional Law* (Mineola, N.Y.: Foundation Press, 1978), 1077–82.

20. Robert Clark, Juanita Kreps, and Joseph Spengler, "Economics of Aging: A Survey," *Journal of Economic Literature* 16 (1978): 929.

21. The federal civil service retirement rules date from the Act of May 22, 1920, 41 Stat. 614, and include the 1978 ADEA Amendments, Pub. L. 95-256, 95 Stat. 189.

22. Derek Parfit, *Reasons and Persons* (Oxford: Oxford University Press, 1986), 319–20.

23. Gordon T. Streib, "Social Stratification and Aging," in *Handbook of Aging and the Social Sciences,* ed. Robert H. Binstock and Ethel Shanas (New York: Van Nostrand Reinhold, 1976), 160.

24. Richard M. Cohn, "Contract and Discrimination" (n.p. 1982), table 2; USDL, *Interim Report to Congress on Age Discrimination,* 10–11.

25. Louis Harris and Associates, Inc., *Aging in the Eighties: America in Transition* (Washington, D.C.: National Council on the Aging, 1981), 47.

26. Erdman Palmore and Kenneth Manton, "Modernization and Status of the Aged: International Correlations," *Journal of Gerontology* 29 (1974): 205; Irwin Press and Mike McKool, Jr., "Social Structure and Status of the Aged: Toward Some Valid Cross-Cultural Generalizations," *Aging and Human Development* 3 (1972): 297.

27. Ernest Watson Burgess, "Aging in Western Culture," in *Aging in Western Societies: A Survey of Social Gerontology,* ed. E. W. Burgess (Chicago: University of Chicago Press, 1960), 3; Donald O. Cowgill, "The Aging of Populations and Societies," *Annals of the American Academy of Political and Social Science* 415 (1974): 1–18; David Gutmann, "The Cross-Cultural Perspective: Notes toward a Comparative Psychology of Aging," in *Handbook of the Psychology of Aging,* ed. James E. Birren and K. Warner Schaie (New York: Van Nostrand Reinhold, 1977), 302; Alexander Mitscherlich, *Society without the Father: A Contribution to Social Psychology,* trans. E. Mosbacher (New York: Schocken, 1970).

28. Geoffrey Gorer, *The American People,* rev. ed. (New York: Norton, 1964).

29. Massachusetts Board of Retirement v. Murgia, 427 U.S. 307 (1976); Vance v. Bradley, 440 U.S. 93 (1979).

30. Murgia v. Massachusetts Board of Retirement, 376 F. Supp. 753, 756 (D. Mass. 1974), *reversed,* 427 U.S. 307 (1976).

31. E.g., Price v. Civil Service Commission [1978] IRLR 291, applying the Sex Discrimination Act of 1975.

Chapter 20.   Empirical Bases of Normative Judgment

1. Lawrence Friedman questions the extent to which the ADEA resulted from normal pressures of lobbying. Lawrence Friedman, *Your Time Will Come: The Law of Age Discrimination and Mandatory Retirement*, Social Research Perspectives, vol. 10 (New York: Russell Sage Foundation, 1984), 16 and n. 39.
2. 78 Stat. 241, 265.
3. U.S. Department of Labor, *The Older American Worker: Age Discrimination in Employment, Report of Secretary of Labor to Congress under Section 715 of Civil Rights Act of 1964* (Washington, D.C.: U.S. Government Printing Office, 1965), 2.
4. 81 Stat. 602, 604.
5. U.S. Department of Labor, Employment Standards Administration, *Age Discrimination in Employment Act of 1967: A Report Covering Activities under the Act during 1976, Submitted to Congress in 1977 in Accordance with Section 13 of the Act* (Washington, D.C.: U.S. Government Printing Office, 1977), 34–37.
6. U.S. Office of Personnel Management, *An Interim Report on the Effects of the Age Discrimination in Employment Act Amendments of 1978 on the Federal Workforce* (Washington, D.C.: U.S. Government Printing Office, 1981).
7. 29 U.S.C.A. §§ 622 and 624 (West Supp. 1987).
8. Grant Gilmore, *The Ages of American Law* (New Haven: Yale University Press, 1977), 99–111.

Epilogue

1. Robert J. Havighurst, "Health Problems in Aging," in *Aging,* ed. Aliza Kolker and Paul I. Ahmed (New York: Elsevier Biomedical, 1982), 141; Thomas McKeown and C. R. Lowe, *An Introduction to Social Medicine* (Oxford: Blackwell Scientific, 1966), 6, 14.
2. Bryan Strong, "History of Aging," in *Aging and the Law Curriculum Materials,* 16, ed. Michael Gilfix (Palo Alto, Calif.: Senior Adults Legal Assistance, 1979): 27–28.
3. The Bible designates each of the holidays of Rosh HaShanah, Yom Kippur, and Sukkot as a *shabbaton,* a recurring period of rest. The sabbatical year is so called in Leviticus 25:4.
4. Abraham P. Block, *The Biblical and Historical Background of Jewish Customs and Ceremonies* (New York: Ktav, 1980), 167.
5. Juanita M. Kreps and Joseph Spengler, "The Leisure Component of Economic Growth," in *Technology and the American Economy,* vol. 2, appendix, "Employment Impact of Technological Change" (Washington, D.C.: U.S. Government Printing Office, 1966).
6. Juanita M. Kreps, "Economics of Retirement," in *Behavior and Adaption in Late Life,* ed. Ewald W. Busse and Eric Pfeiffer (Boston: Little, Brown, 1969).

7. Juanita M. Kreps, *Lifetime Allocation of Work and Income: Essays in the Economics of Aging* (Durham, N.C.: Duke University Press, 1971), 21–22.
8. Juanita M. Kreps, "Time for Leisure, Time for Work," *Monthly Labor Review* 92 (April 1969): 60–61.
9. The Age Discrimination in Employment Act includes an education and research program, 29 U.S.C. 621(a)(3) (1982).
10. U.S. Department of Labor, *The Older American Worker: Age Discrimination in Employment, Report of Secretary of Labor to Congress under Section 715 of Civil Rights Act of 1964* (Washington, D.C.: U.S. Government Printing Office, 1965).
11. Anna-Stina Ericson, "The Employment of Older Workers Abroad," *Monthly Labor Review* 83 (March 1960): 274.
12. 29 U.S.C.A. § 626(d) (West Supp. 1987).
13. 29 U.S.C.A. § 623(f)(1) (West Supp. 1987).
14. Vance v. Bradley, 440 U.S. 93, 108–9, 111–12.
15. Massachusetts Board of Retirement v. Murgia, 427 U.S. 307, 312 (1976); Vance v. Bradley, 440 U.S. 93, 97–98 (1979).
16. *Murgia,* 427 U.S. at 311.
17. William Graebner, *A History of Retirement: The Meaning and Function of an American Institution, 1885–1978* (New Haven: Yale University Press, 1980).
18. Sir James George Frazer, *The Golden Bough: A Study in Magic and Religion* (1850), 3d ed. (London: Macmillan, 1926) pt. 1, "The Magic Art and the Evolution of Kings," 1:8–9.
19. Ibid., vii.
20. Sigmund Freud, "Totem and Taboo" (1913–14), in *The Standard Edition of the Complete Psychological Works of Sigmund Freud,* ed. and trans. James Strachey (London: Hogarth, 1975), vol. 13.

Index

223

About the author

Martin Lyon Levine, J.D., is the UPS Foundation Professor of Law, Gerontology, Psychiatry and the Behavioral Sciences at the University of Southern California and director of the Oxford-USC Institute of Legal Theory. He is president of the International Society of Aging, Law and Ethics and has been general counsel of the U.S. Senate Constitutional Rights Subcommittee.